Activity Analysis, Creativity, and Playfulness in Pediatric Occupational Therapy

Making Play Just Right

Heather Miller Kuhaneck, MS, OTR/L

CLINICAL ASSISTANT PROFESSOR, SACRED HEART UNIVERSITY

Susan L. Spitzer, PhD, OTR/L

PRIVATE PRACTICE

Elissa Miller, OTD, OTR/L

ASSISTANT PROFESSOR, SACRED HEART UNIVERSITY

JONES AND BARTLETT PUBLISHERS

Sudbury, Massachusetts

BOSTON   TORONTO   LONDON   SINGAPORE

World Headquarters
Jones and Bartlett Publishers
40 Tall Pine Drive
Sudbury, MA 01776
978-443-5000
info@jbpub.com
www.jbpub.com

Jones and Bartlett Publishers Canada
6339 Ormindale Way
Mississauga, Ontario L5V 1J2
Canada

Jones and Bartlett Publishers International
Barb House, Barb Mews
London W6 7PA
United Kingdom

Jones and Bartlett's books and products are available through most bookstores and online booksellers. To contact Jones and Bartlett Publishers directly, call 800-832-0034, fax 978-443-8000, or visit our website, www.jbpub.com.

Substantial discounts on bulk quantities of Jones and Bartlett's publications are available to corporations, professional associations, and other qualified organizations. For details and specific discount information, contact the special sales department at Jones and Bartlett via the above contact information or send an email to specialsales@jbpub.com.

The authors, editor, and publisher have made every effort to provide accurate information. However, they are not responsible for errors, omissions, or for any outcomes related to the use of the contents of this book and take no responsibility for the use of the products and procedures described. Treatments and side effects described in this book may not be applicable to all people; likewise, some people may require a dose or experience a side effect that is not described herein. Drugs and medical devices are discussed that may have limited availability controlled by the Food and Drug Administration (FDA) for use only in a research study or clinical trial. Research, clinical practice, and government regulations often change the accepted standard in this field. When consideration is being given to use of any drug in the clinical setting, the healthcare provider or reader is responsible for determining FDA status of the drug, reading the package insert, and reviewing prescribing information for the most up-to-date recommendations on dose, precautions, and contraindications, and determining the appropriate usage for the product. This is especially important in the case of drugs that are new or seldom used.

Production Credits

Publisher: David Cella
Acquisitions Editor: Kristine Jones
Associate Editor: Maro Gartside
Production Assistant: Laura Almozara
Manufacturing and Inventory Control Supervisor: Amy Bacus

Composition: Spoke & Wheel/Jason Miranda
Assistant Photo Researcher: Meghan Hayes
Cover Design: Scott Moden
Printing and Binding: Courier Kendallville
Cover Printing: Courier Kendallville

Cover Images

Front Cover
Girl with bear and stethoscope: © Jaimie Duplass/ShutterStock, Inc.
Little boy, truck, blocks: © Olgysha/ShutterStock, Inc.
Baby sitting with blocks: © Flashon Studio/ShutterStock, Inc
Woman, two boys at table: © matka_Wariatka/ShutterStock, Inc.
Boy, soccer ball: © Monkey Business Images/ShutterStock, Inc.
Two girls, painting: © Thomas M. Perkins/ShutterStock, Inc.

Spine
Smiling girl: © Jacek Chabraszewski/ShutterStock, Inc.

Back Cover
Girl, blocks: © Dagmara Ponikiewska/ShutterStock, Inc.

Library of Congress Cataloging-in-Publication Data

Miller Kuhaneck, Heather.
   Activity analysis, creativity, and playfulness in pediatric occupational therapy : making play just right / Heather Miller Kuhaneck, Susan L. Spitzer, Elissa Miller.
      p. ; cm.
   Includes bibliographical references and index.
   ISBN-13: 978-0-7637-5606-2 (alk. paper)
   ISBN-10: 0-7637-5606-7 (alk. paper)
   1. Occupational therapy for children. 2. Play therapy. I. Spitzer, Susan L. II. Miller, Elissa. III. Title.
   [DNLM: 1. Occupational Therapy—methods. 2. Play Therapy—methods. 3. Child. 4. Developmental Disabilities—rehabilitation. 5. Disabled Children—rehabilitation. WS 350.2 M6487a 2010]
   RJ53.O25M55 2010
   618.92'89165—dc22
                                          2009012406

6048
Printed in the United States of America
14 13 12   10 9 8 7 6 5 4

Brief Contents

Contents

SECTION THREE   . . .And How to Apply Them   95

CHAPTER 5   Selecting Play Activities: Activity Analysis,
Clinical Reasoning, and Frames of Reference   97

CHAPTER 6   Adapting Play Activities   *113*

CHAPTER 7   Creating Therapeutic Play Activities   *127*

Preface

A core tenet of this book is that the meaning of the activities we engage in with our clients is the key to intervention effectiveness. For a pediatric client, the primary meaningful occupation is play. Therefore, for pediatric occupational therapy to be maximally effective, we believe that it is our professional responsibility to incorporate play into our interventions with children.

In our experience, we noted the difficulty students and novice therapists have in applying activity analysis to pediatric interventions to create a fluid, playful atmosphere. Most writings about activity analysis focus on adult interventions and adult examples. It is our hope that by guiding the application of activity analysis to playful pediatric intervention, we may assist occupational therapists in more clearly practicing client-centered, occupation-focused pediatric therapy.

This book, like many projects that span a long period of time, evolved and changed as it emerged into the form you read today. The initial focus of the book, using activity analysis in pediatric intervention, morphed and changed as our commitment to a playful approach to therapy took center stage. What you see now is the result of a true collaboration among three very playful adults and teachers who want to encourage others to join in our fun.

The book provides the background, history, evidence, and general knowledge needed to use the approach we recommend as well as the specific examples and recommendations needed to help therapists adopt these strategies. Additionally, we provide a number of case examples and companion videos to allow the reader to engage in learning activities to improve understanding of the content. We believe the videos to be especially important as we all collectively value the experiences we have had being mentored while we observed a master clinician treating. Although it is impossible to ensure every therapist gets that opportunity, by demonstrating key principles within videotaped intervention sessions, it is our hope that the skills and strategies will come alive and be more readily understood and adopted.

Although the information we present is substantiated by research where research exists, it is also supported by our combined 40 years of pediatric practice using a play-based approach. Each of us has been guided by the work of A. Jean Ayres, and we are all lucky to have been mentored by those who are experts in practice. We all strongly believe in the need for mentoring in practice and hope that this book will be just one facet of your learning, learning that will be applied in practice with a mentor.

In keeping with the content of the text, we have tried to maintain a playful and somewhat informal writing style. We hope that the style, content, and format allow you to enjoy your learning experience as you progress through this text. As you read and practice the strategies suggested in this book, we hope you have fun and truly experience the power of play.

Acknowledgments

Completing any body of work requires the collaborative efforts of many individuals, and this text is no exception. We would like to specifically thank the following people for their contributions and assistance: Maro Gartside for her patience and assistance with our endless questions and queries; Chris Marrs for his time and expertise in video editing; the numerous friends, family, and clients who agreed to be photographed and videotaped; our clients throughout the years, as each one has taught and inspired us, and that cumulative experience is reflected and embedded in these pages; and our colleagues who have encouraged and helped us by reviewing drafts of this text. Finally, we of course each need to acknowledge the sacrifice of our families, who allowed us the time to devote to this creative enterprise and labor of love.

There is nothing that screams "PLAY" to me more than watching my two dogs, Kramer and Abigail, totally in the moment romping through the woods on our hikes, and their playful nature energizes mine. So, I must recognize their sacrifice, as over the past year they often had to cheerfully wait for me to finish my work before we could go out to play. Well, maybe they weren't so cheerful about it but they learned to wait if not to understand. More importantly, to my husband, Shayne, my enduring love and gratitude. Your playful, silly side helps keep me sane when I become too serious, and your steady support and encouragement allows me to grow.

—*HMK*

To my friends and family, I am so grateful for your understanding, patience, and humor. Together we have forgone so much as I put lots of play on hold to work on this book. Most of all, to my husband, David Morales, my love, gratitude, and admiration for you are only deepened by your enduring sacrifices and support. You have given up the most on a daily basis and yet have remained my greatest supporter, always believing in me even when I doubt myself. The moments of playfulness and silliness on which you insist are a welcome respite from work and the reminder I needed of the play that awaits me now. Thank you.

—*SLS*

My deepest love and thanks to my husband, Todd, the most fun and playful grown man I know. I will never forget your patience and willingness to support and encourage me during this process. To my two little play "monsters," Ethan and Perry, I love you and cherish every moment we spend together. You are my true inspiration for this work.

—*EM*

Reviewers

Christine Achenbach, MEd, OTR/L
Fieldwork Coordinator
Department of Occupational Therapy
Elizabethtown College
Elizabethtown, PA

M. Irma Alvarado, PhD, OTR/L
Associate Professor
Occupational Therapy Department
Brenau University
Gainesville, GA

Jody Bortone, EdD, OTR/L
Chair and Director
Graduate Program in Occupational
  Therapy
Sacred Heart University
Fairfield, CT

Judy Beck Ericksen, PhD, OTR/L
Associate Professor
Department of Occupational Therapy
Elizabethtown College
Elizabethtown, PA

Cynthia Haynes, MEd, MBA, OTR/L
Associate Professor
Occupational Therapy Program
Academic Clinical Education Coordinator
Philadelphia University
Philadelphia, PA

Lynn Jaffe, ScD, OTR/L
Associate Professor
Department of Occupational Therapy
Medical College of Georgia
Augusta, GA

Diane Parham, PhD, OTR/L, FAOTA
Professor and Director
Occupational Therapy Graduate Program
University of New Mexico
Albuquerque, NM

Susan B. Young, MA, OTD, OTR/L, FAOTA
Associate Professor
School of Occupational Therapy
Belmont University
Nashville, TN

Section One
The Knowledge You Need...

1

The Who, What, Where, When, and Why of Play

After reading this chapter the reader will

1. Recognize the universality of play across the globe and across species.

2. Compare and contrast play and playfulness.

3. Describe the characteristics of play.

4. Describe the multiple influences on children's play choices and play places.

5. Identify the typical patterns of development of play in humans.

6. Summarize theories of why children play.

> *Play is training for the unexpected.*
> —Mark Bekoff

A substantial body of work exists describing the many theories and beliefs about why we play, documenting the developmental processes that occur in the play of children and establishing that humans are not the only creatures that participate in this activity. New information about play, garnered through the study of species other than humans as well as through the ability to examine the brain in new ways, has increasingly justified the importance of play. This chapter forms the backbone for the following chapters on playful intervention in this text, providing an overview of that literature and an explanation of our commitment to play in our practice. This knowledge base is crucial to inform therapeutic reasoning when analyzing and promoting play and consulting with clients regarding the nuances and complexities of play. In this chapter we answer the "w" questions of play: Who plays, what is play, what do children play, when does play occur, where does play occur, and why do children play?

■ WHO PLAYS?

Play is often considered something that only children do. However, adolescents and adults play as well. Play may look different in the infant, young child, teen, or adult, but play of some form occurs in most all individuals depending on how you define or describe play. Some use different terms for play at various ages; for example, the word "play" is used primarily for the activities of infants, toddlers, and children, whereas "recreation" or "leisure" is the term often used for adults (Sutton-Smith, 1997). If one uses recreation or leisure for the play of adults, then one could say adults do not "play." Adults, however, are certainly capable of play, and some adults are in fact quite playful. However, many adults are not taught how to play with children and, if not raised themselves with playful parents, may not actively seek to engage in play with children (Singer & Singer, 1992, 2001).

Most all children play. There is evidence of a variety of toys and games indicating that children have played throughout history since the ancient Greeks, Sumerians, and Egyptians (Barnes, 2006). Children in both modern societies and hunter-gatherer societies play (Gosso et al., 2005; Kamei, 2005). Children across the globe in diverse cultures play. Both homeless children and even children in refugee camps can and do play (Boxill & Beaty, 1990; Harrington & Dawson, 1997; Scarlett, Naudeau, Salonius-Pasternak, & Ponte, 2005).[1] Children with disabilities also play, although children with severe cognitive

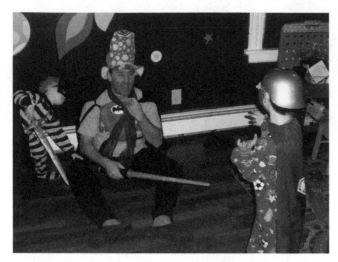

Some adults are quite playful.

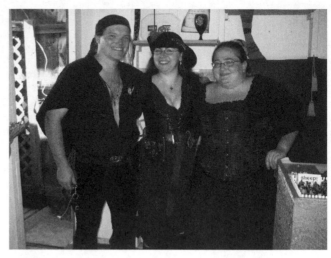

Many adults still enjoy dressing up.

disabilities may not demonstrate all forms of play. Some research has suggested that play may be limited or absent in children who later grow into violent adults (S. Brown, 1998, Brown, 2006). Play therefore appears to be a universal aspect of *typical* child development.

In addition to humans of all ages, nonhuman species play too. Dogs play, cats play, and rodents play, and elaborate play has been observed in both ravens and primates (Bekoff & Byers, 1998; Burghart, 2005; Heinrich & Smolker, 1998). Play has been observed even in turtles, lizards, and fish (Burghart, 2005). Because play is observed in all orders of mammals, play probably exists in even the earliest mammals to evolve (Burghart, 1984, 2005). Similar to the human species, play is primarily observed in juvenile animals, and often juveniles are each other's preferred play partners. However, when no juveniles are available, adult primates will play with their young just as adult humans often do (Biben, 1998).

Some believe that human play is different because humans pretend. However, pretend play may be more related to language ability than species. In primates who have been trained to use language, there is some evidence of pretend play (Gomes & Martin-Andrade, 2005). Chimps who have learned sign language have been noted to pretend with dolls, and Koko the gorilla, who also signs, has been noted to play with dolls as well. Although pretense is not pervasive and symbolism is not typical in apes, these language-trained primates may be in a "zone of proximal evolution"[2] (Gomes & Martin-Andrade, 2005).

These differences between the play of humans and nonhumans and between adults and children lead us nicely into the discussion of the difficulty in defining play. Is it play when a gorilla carries a doll? Is it play when dogs chase a stick? Is it play when adults are interacting with children in a game and are purposely limiting their own abilities to make the game more fair and even for the child? Just what is play anyway?

■ WHAT IS PLAY?

The word "play" is used in multiple fashions and has many connotations. Early usage of the term often was related to motion, for example, the motion of the fingers in "playing" a musical instrument (Burghart, 2005). People use the word "play" as a noun, as in the dramatic theater productions put on stage. People can also use the word to discuss

---

[1] "Play is now understood to be one of the most effective ways of helping children living in the aftermath of disasters and the midst of wars to begin healing" (Murphy, 2005). Additionally, play is recognized as a child's right across the globe. Article 31 of the United Nation's *Convention on the Rights of the Child* (1989) states, "Parties recognize the right of the child to rest and leisure, to engage in play and recreational activities appropriate to the age of the child and to participate freely in cultural life and the arts." A multitude of countries (193 thus far) have ratified this document (see *http://www.unhchr.ch/pdf/report.pdf*). Once signed, a country is bound by international law to adopt the document's human rights protections for children, including the right to play. Sadly, the United States has not yet ratified this document (see *http://childrightscampaign.org/crcindex.php*). However, the American Occupational Therapy Association has issued a statement affirming a child's right to play (see *http://www.aota.org/News/Media/Statements/41043.aspx*).

[2] The term "zone of proximal evolution" is adapted from the work of Vygotsky (1978) from "zone of proximal development" described later in the chapter.

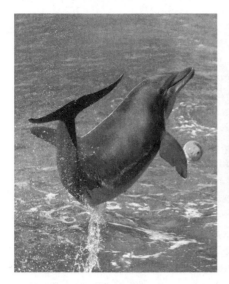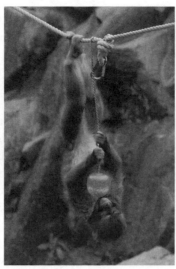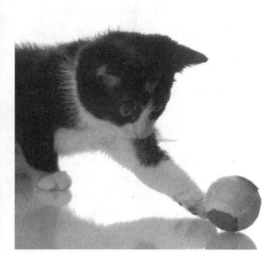

Most mammals play.

sensory experiences, as in observing the "play" of light on the surface of the ocean. Modern usage of the word "play" in terms of children's behavior suggests an activity that is "spirited, voluntary and fun" (Burghart, 2005, p. 23). People can also play dead, play the radio, play with food, play it safe, or make a play for something.

Many have attempted to define the word "play," and we begin with their examples. Huizinga (1955) was an early author who described play as something occurring for its own sake. His definition stated that play was fully absorbing, included some element of uncertainty, involved illusion or exaggeration, and was clearly not real to those doing it. Fagan (1984) defined play as "performance . . . of active behavioral interactions that enable the player to adjust to and create its own environment, both ecological and social" (p. 169). Sutton-Smith (1997) defined play as novel adaptation similar to the evolutionary struggle for survival. Burghart (2005) suggested this definition, which could encompass both animal play and human play: "Play is repeated, incompletely functional behavior differing from more serious versions structurally, contextually, or ontogenetically, and initiated voluntarily when the animal is in a relaxed or low stress setting" (p. 82). Some authors define play very broadly in the way children define play, as "almost anything enjoyable" (Scarlett et al., 2005, p. 4). Similarly, the National Institute for Play defines play as "a state of being that is intensely pleasurable. It energizes and enlivens us. It eases our burdens, renews a natural sense of optimism and opens us up to new possibilities."[3] Each of these definitions works for some or

many forms of play, but not all. The play of humans is difficult to define concisely, but people generally believe they know it when they see it.

The idea that play is more of an *attitude* than a *thing* has been considered as well. Playfulness as an attitude or a disposition appears easier to define and measure (Barnett, 1990). Many authors have worked at both defining playfulness and creating measures of it (Barnett, 1990, 1991; Lieberman, 1965, 1966; Skard & Bundy, 2008). Millar (1968) suggested that playfulness is about creative possibilities and removing constraints. Rubin, Fein, and Vandenberg (1983) suggested that play could be defined with three dimensions: disposition, behavior, and contexts. Considering the importance of the playful attitude for play, Ferland (2005) defined play as a subjective attitude in which pleasure, interest, and spontaneity are combined and that is expressed through freely chosen behavior where no specific performance is expected. The criteria used for many of these authors included the motivation source, goal orientation, degree of stimuli domination, flexibility, affect, rule boundaries, and active involvement of the person observed. Each of these aspects occurred in degrees, and, as the relative combination of them increased, an activity was more likely to be described as playful or play (Rogers et al., 1998).

Although there is some consensus regarding the characteristics of play (see **Figure 1-1**), differences of opinion do exist. As reminded by Sutton-Smith and Kelly-Byrne (1984), play can often be idealized by adults in Western cultures. For example, not all play is fun. Some play is scary. Play can be dangerous and risky. Some play is cruel, and children are left out. Play can be about struggles

[3] see *http://www.nifplay.org/front_door.html*

Learning Activities

1. Think about the words and the concepts of play and playfulness. How are they similar and different? Can you compare and contrast the two terms?

2. In lieu of trying to create one definition that captures play, many authors have instead generated lists of characteristics that describe play. There is typically consensus regarding the characteristics included in such lists, and the words "fun" or "pleasurable" often top the lists. Consider the list of characteristics in **Figure 1-1** that play activities demonstrate. Does the list seem to capture all forms of play?

---

for power and dominance. Sometimes play is not voluntary; children often must defer to more powerful or dominant children. Some play is highly sexualized. And not all play is free and flexible; some play is highly rule bound and structured (Sutton-Smith & Kelly-Byrne, 1984). Thus lists of characteristics of play help, but even with these lists, there is not complete consensus.

Reilly (1974) likened the task of defining play to "defining a cobweb" and stated, "only the naïve could believe from reviewing the evidence of the literature that play is a behavior having an identifiable nature. While common sense may confidently assert that there is such a thing as play, the literature assumes a rather weak position about what this phenomenon is" (p. 113). Burghart (2005) similarly suggested that the problems with defining play are "legendary" (p. 49).

Figure 1-1   Common Characteristics of Activities Defined as Play

- Flexibility
- Spontaneity
- Intrinsic motivation
- Nonliteral or symbolic use of objects
- Voluntary engagement
- Free choice
- Elicitation of positive affect (fun/enjoyable)
- Lack of functional purpose or goal
- Often resembles real behaviors but lacks the consequences

Information compiled by the authors from a variety of sources cited in this chapter

However, here we offer a definition of play to provide a shared understanding for this book. For the purposes of this book, we state that *play is any activity freely entered into that is fun or enjoyable and that is appropriately matched to one's skill to represent an attainable challenge.* Our definition is similar to others in the literature but different from many as well. We have included each portion of this definition for specific reasons. For example, the inclusion of fun and enjoyment is intended to give voice to the importance and meaning of play as described by children themselves. If play is defined as children define play, play is fun (Heah, Case, McGuire, & Law, 2007; Miller & Kuhaneck, 2008; Scarlett et al., 2005; Wiltz & Fein, 2006). Using "fun" in our definition of play, however, provides us with yet another dilemma. "If we could come up with a workable definition of fun and measure it objectively, we would still be left with the begging question 'why is this particular behavior fun?'" (Heinrich & Smolker, 1998, p. 28). For many children and adults, fun means that the game or toy provides an appropriate level of challenge (Ayres, 1979, 2005; Csikszentmihalyi, 1990; Miller & Kuhaneck, 2008; Vygotsky, 1978). Therefore our definition captures the importance of the "just right challenge" for play to be fun. This concept of the need for the "just right challenge" (Ayres, 1979, 2005) in play is one we explore later in the chapter and throughout the book. Finally, the idea of play as voluntary and freely entered into is included because of the literature on the importance of intrinsic motivation for fun and play. Thus someone else may suggest or structure play, but the child is intrinsically motivated to participate. This definition is purposefully broad to allow us to encompass the range of play of children with disabilities and particularly those with autism, as well as the sport and leisure of teenagers. Speaking of this range of play then brings us to the next topic: What are the different types of play?

Question: What is play?

Answer: Play is any activity freely entered into that is fun or enjoyable and that is appropriately matched to one's skill to represent an attainable challenge.

What Are the Different Types of Play?

Often, because of the difficulty defining and explaining play as one large construct, play has been divided into different categories or types. Some authors have divided play simply into two categories, play and exploration, whereas others have created elaborate lists of multiple forms of play behaviors. Often, the categories of play behaviors follow developmental sequences and thus intermingle play forms with developmental achievements. Just a few of the categorization schemes are provided here as examples to familiarize the reader with this terminology for later sections of the chapter.

Some separate exploratory behaviors and play (Burghart, 2005; Hutt, 1966), stating that exploratory behaviors occur with novel objects and allow the child to determine the properties of the object, whereas play emerges once the child understands the object and then seeks to determine what he or she can *do* with it. Others find this distinction less important. For example, Power (2000) suggested that perhaps a category halfway between the two is needed that corresponds to the combination of play and exploration that often co occurs.

There are many other descriptions of play types; one older categorization of play created by Belsky and Most (1981) lists 11 different types of play (**Figure 1-2**). Others suggest play can simply be categorized as social or nonsocial, or symbolic (pretend) or nonsymbolic/sensorimotor. McGhee (1984) makes a distinction between play that is interesting but not humorous, and playful play, which has elements of humor and incongruity. Power (2000) lists five categories of play: locomotor, solitary object, social object/pretend, play fighting, and parent–child play. Bateson (2005) lists solitary, imaginative, symbolic, verbal, social, constructive, manipulative, and rough and tumble as forms or categories of play. Finally, a recent categorization scheme from the National Institute for Play[4] suggests seven types or patterns of play (see **Figure 1-3**). Although the categories described by the National Institute for Play fit nicely with the broad scope of occupational therapy, these categories have not been widely used thus far in the literature. One can see how over time, the thinking regarding types of play has changed, and one can see how certain categorization schemes intertwine with developmental patterns.

Consequently, for the purposes of this chapter—to clearly report the body of knowledge that exists in the realm of play preferences and play development—we use

Figure 1-2   Categories of Play

- Mouthing play
- Simple manipulation play
- Functional play (objects are manipulated appropriately)
- Relational play (objects are combined in a nonfunctional fashion, e.g., putting a toy banana on a doll bed)
- Functional-relational play (objects are combined appropriately, e.g., a toy banana on a toy plate or a baby doll on a toy bed)
- Enactive naming play (pretend without confirmation, such as when a young toddler places the play phone to his head without making any sounds)
- Pretend self-play (pretend activity on oneself, e.g., pretending to eat a toy banana)
- Pretend play other (pretending to feed a baby doll)
- Substitution play (using one object in pretend for another, e.g., using the toy banana as a telephone)
- Sequence pretend play (linked pretend schemes such as feeding the baby, then putting it to bed)
- Sequenced substitution play (same as sequenced play but with an object substitution)

Adapted from Belsky & Most, 1981

Figure 1-3   Seven Patterns of Play

- *Attunement play:* emotional and interactive play with caregivers
- *Body play and movement:* movement-related play that helps a child learn about the body
- *Object play:* play with toys and objects
- *Social play:* rough and tumble play, celebratory play
- *Imaginative and pretend play:* symbolic play
- *Storytelling and narrative play:* telling of or acting out of stories
- *Transformative-integrative and creative play:* play through the imagination, allowing creativity to emerge

Adapted from *http://www.nifplay.org/science_intro.html*

Question: What are the different types of play?

Answer: It depends on whom you ask. We like the categories described by the National Institute for Play.

[4] see *http://www.nifplay.org/science_intro.html*

the variety of play labels as they have been used by different authors in the past.

■ WHAT DO CHILDREN LIKE TO PLAY?

The toys children play with and the play activities children enjoy have changed over time. Evidence of early playthings suggests ancient and early peoples played with dolls, balls, rattles, drums, hobby horses, toy "men" or soldiers, games with rules, puzzles, and construction toys (Barnes, 2006). Although many of these toys and games remain, the advent of a variety of commercially available, technologically sophisticated toys has allowed new forms of play to emerge, such as video game play. In addition, changes in society and toy availability have also limited previously common play (Christakis, Ebel, Rivara, & Zimmerman, 2004; Levin & Rosenquest, 2001; Media Analysis Laboratory, 1998; Rivkin, 2006; Singer & Singer, 2001). Children today are less likely to play outside and generally spend more time in sedentary play (Clements, 2004; Rivkin, 2006; Singer & Singer, 2001) and children are much more likely to play with electronic toys and other digital media (Elkind, 2001; Singer & Singer, 2001).

Research throughout the past hundred years has carefully described the activities children like to play. The large body of literature allows us to make some generalizations regarding children's play preferences. First, children's play preferences change with age and the development of new skills. Second, children's play preferences vary by gender, although it is still unclear to what extent this is a function of biology or culture. Finally, children's preferences are influenced by the physical and sociocultural environment in which they live and play. Although the *content* of preferred play may have changed over time, development and gender appear to be stable factors influencing play preferences (Case-Smith & Miller Kuhaneck, 2008; Miller & Kuhaneck, 2008).

Age and Development

As children grow and learn, they progress through stages and exhibit different play behaviors (Benjamin, 1932; Cole & LaVoie, 1985; Fein, 1981; Garner & Bergen, 2006; Johnson, 2006; Lowe, 1975; Manning, 2006; Parten, 1932; Pellegrini, 2006; Piaget, 1962; Takata, 1974). Many authors have written about specific sequences in play development; one of the most familiar may be Piaget's cognitive levels in regard to play (Piaget, 1952/1972, 1962).

Piaget's stages are the sensorimotor stage, the preoperational stage, the stage of concrete operations, and the stage of formal operations. In the sensorimotor stage, the infant's reflexive behaviors eventually grow into independent interaction with the environment. The infant's sensorimotor behaviors become more intentional and more refined. Through processes of assimilation and accommodation, the infant learns about the world and begins to solve simple problems. By 2 years of age the toddler begins to use mental representation and begins more social interactions. Language skills grow during this period, and the child can use sensorimotor behaviors to solve problems. The child over time begins to have moral reasoning and eventually becomes focused on rules. From ages 7 to 11 years, the child is developing logical thought and can solve most concrete problems. During the next stage, the child's ability to think abstractly grows and emerges, and the child can use logic for an argument or to solve hypothetical problems. When considering Piaget's stages of cognitive development, one views the development of play as intertwined with cognitive development (Piaget, 1952/1975, 1962).

In infancy, play begins to emerge and differentiate from exploration (Garner & Bergen, 2006; Piaget, 1952, 1962). Actions that occur by chance begin to be repeated purposely. In play, the infant learns what he or she can do with objects and body parts that provide enjoyment. In this infant stage, the enjoyment received is typically sensory in nature, although enjoyment can occur from social interactions as well. Because infants cannot tell people when they are playing or not playing, adults infer this from their cues. Infant cues for play include smiles, giggles, positive affect, and the desire for repetition of a motion or action. As infants grow and develop, imitative abilities

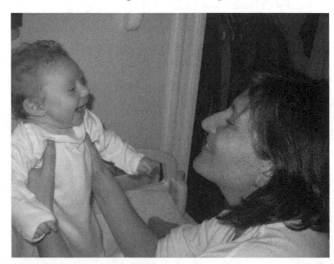

Infant social play and positive affect.

begin to figure prominently in play, and simple turn-taking emerges. Infants learn from adults to read play from non-play and over time learn to invent their own games and provide cues to others to signal that what they are doing is also play. These skills of reading play cues begin early in infancy with games like "peekaboo," and by the second year of life, children are creating their own games with their own play cues (Garner & Bergen, 2006).

Object play and sensorimotor play predominates at young ages. Noticeable preferences for specific objects may be observed as early as 3 months of age, although a favorite toy is indicated by less than 50% of infants that young (Furby & Wilke, 1982). Closer to 90% of infants prefer one favored object by 1 year of age (Furby &

Wilke, 1982). Object play progresses from single-object use to combined object play (Gowen, Johnson-Martin, Goldman, & Hussey, 1992). Single-object play is seen in infancy and decreases from 7 to 18 months of age as the child begins to combine objects in greater frequency. Object play also progresses from use of an object indiscriminately to the use of an object in a way that demonstrates understanding of its unique features (Gowen et al., 1992). Early object play is sensorimotor in nature, with much mouthing, banging, and waving. Later object play involves using objects as they are intended. Children about 1 year of age investigate and explore new objects primarily, but by 15 months, discriminative play is more common (Garner & Bergen, 2006).

The second year of life is important as symbolic play begins to take hold. As the child matures, symbolic play and more complex pretense and role play emerge (Fein, 1981; Gowen et al., 1992). Pretend play expands from simple pretense, such as talking into a play phone, to more complex pretense, such as feeding a baby doll. Initially, a child requires props for pretense, and early props must look quite real. Over time, the need for these replicas

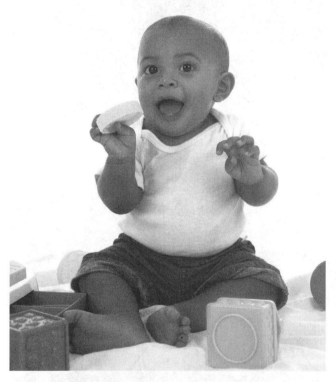

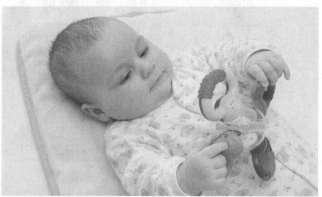

Early infant play is exploratory and manipulative.

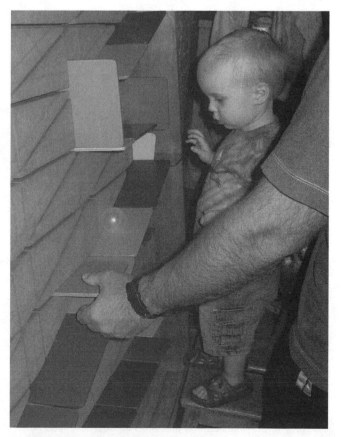

Toddlers enjoy play that combines objects.

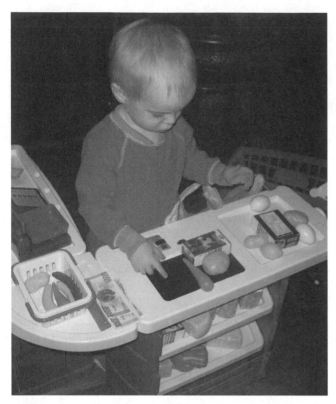

Pretend play flourishes initially with realistic props.

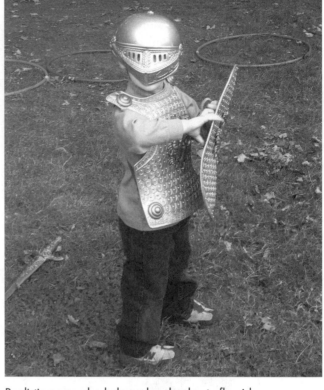

Realistic props also help early role play to flourish.

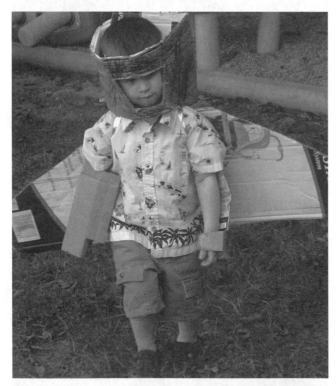

Pretend play does not require expensive commercial props—a variety of costumes can be made from household materials.

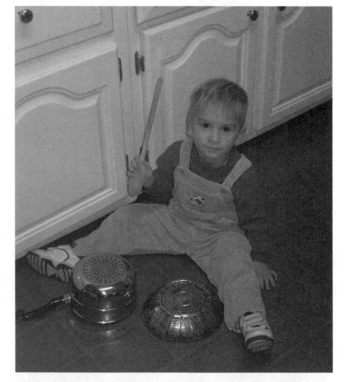

Eventually props do not need to look very realistic—these pots, pans, and spoons serve quite well as drums for the preschool-age child.

diminishes and objects can be substituted for other objects. Eventually, props are not needed as a child imagines their existence while playing (Garner & Bergen, 2006).

The preschool period brings with it greater language abilities and a significant emphasis on pretend play (Fein, 1981). Children of this age often pretend with toys of a variety of media, for example, creating pretend games while completing a puzzle or building with Legos. Pretend play can occur while drawing or painting or while climbing on a structure in a playground. Pretend play is often strongly connected with emotions and feelings. Children act out experiences they have had and desires that they cannot actually experience outside of play. Pretend play is also more and more social as children age (Garner & Bergen, 2006; Johnson, 2006).

With the increase in the social aspects of pretense, the ability to read and send cues is crucial because pretend actions often can look identical to the real action. How do people know a child is pretending? They must infer from the behaviors; they see facial expressions, smiles, different eye gaze, and positive affect. Contextual cues may help as well, such as a child pretending to be asleep in a location

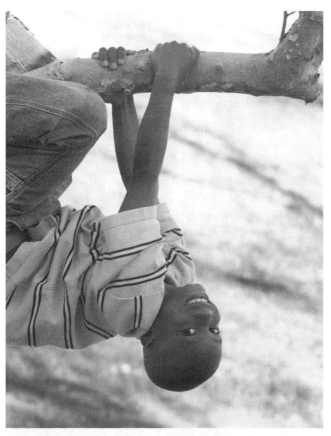

Throughout early childhood, active play is a preferred form and children often seek to defy or challenge gravity.

where he or she would not normally be sleeping. Generally, a child who is pretending may wish to take turns in the "game" with another. These contextual cues assist adults in the determination that the child is playing (Garner & Bergen, 2006).

Preschool also brings a greater level of activity (Halverson & Waldrop, 1973; Pellegrini & Smith, 1998a/b, 2003) and a variety of gross motor and playground play that appears sensory seeking in nature. Preschool-age children love to swing, spin, run, climb, hang, jump, and be upside down (Chew, 1985; Sandseter, 2007). Why is movement so important for young children? While the vestibular apparatus is fully formed at birth, functionally it continues to develop for many years as children move, explore, and play (Cherng, Chen, & Su, 2001; Lai & Chan, 2002). These sensory-rich activities that children engage in during preschool correspond with significant new motor skills as children learn to balance on one foot, hop, skip, gallop, and challenge gravity.

Elementary school-age children play somewhat differently (Johnson, 2006). In school, pretend play diminishes as peer play increasingly occurs outside the classroom on the playground and is made up of more physical or social games. Boys tend to engage in rough and tumble play, whereas girls tend to engage in games such as jump-rope, rhyming games, and other social forms of play. Pretending still may occur in the home or after school. Pretend play during this period is quite complex and often more tied to reality than it was in preschool. For example, children may pretend to be famous singers. The amount of preparation that goes into play during this stage is substantial. Younger children just want to play, whereas older children want to properly set the stage (Johnson, 2006).

Games with rules emerge as very important to both genders. Board games and video games become very popular. During this time, children often play with peers with collections of items and trading games. Large amounts of negotiation can occur in the attempt for children to grow their collections. These games with rules can require elaborate planning and preparation as the children establish what the rules are. Competition and collaboration can become more emphasized in both genders as children engage in more team competitive sports (Johnson, 2006; Piaget, 1962).

Aggressive-themed play and true aggression in play also can emerge during this time period (Blurton Jones, 1978). Wrestling, soldiers, space warriors, pirates, and super heroes are common themes where a form of aggression arises. This form of play appears to be universal

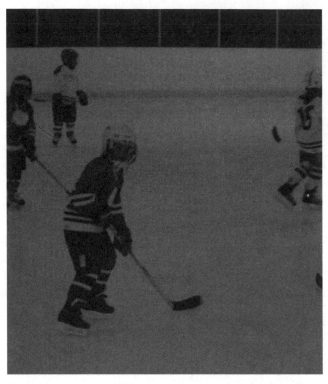

Sports and other games with rules predominate during the elementary years.

but is influenced by cultural norms. In cultures where aggression is less tolerated, the play fighting includes more chase and flee games and less aggressive rough and tumble play (Fry, 2005). These culturally defined judgments about whether aggressive play is acceptable are not yet supported by research to determine the benefits or detriments of such play. Power (2000) suggested that rough and tumble play may have positive functions for children in general but may be detrimental for overly aggressive or rejected children. Play fighting is only correlated with real aggression for children who are rejected by their peers but not for children in general (Pellegrini, 1988, 1994). Various adaptive functions have been proposed for this form of play, such as the development of aggression prevention and control, social relationships, and flexibility in handling social problems (Blurton Jones, 1978; Glassner, 1976; Goldstein, 1995; Pellegrini, 1995; Power, 2000). Play fighting may provide an acceptable excuse for physical contact and opportunities to care for each other (e.g., helping someone get up and checking if that person is okay, etc. (Reed, 2005). It may also provide a sense of excitement as long as there is confidence that the players are in a safe environment (Apter, 1991). Play fighting may be beneficial at younger ages but may morph into something dangerous if it continues into adolescent bullying. Some

teens do use rough and tumble play as a way to exert their dominance (Pellegrini, 2006).

In adolescence, play changes in other ways as well, and teens tend to spend much of their time socializing with peers (Cummings & Vandewater, 2007; Gordon & Caltabiano, 1996; Pawelko & Magafas, 1997; Zill, Winquist Nord, & Loomis, 1995). Common teen forms of play or leisure include formal and informal sports, video game play, watching movies with friends, and talking on the telephone or texting. However, often the leisure time of teens is spent in risky, unproductive, or sedentary behaviors. Given the potential link between adolescent leisure patterns and the leisure patterns of adults and the possible impact of playful adult leisure and psychological health, the importance of a well-balanced and active play leisure profile in adolescence seems clear (Hektner & Csikszentmihalyi, 1996; Scott & Willits, 1998; Staempfli, 2007).

The changes in play seen with children's cognitive, social-emotional, and physical development are clear. Does play drive development or merely reflect it? We believe that development and play together grow in a spiraling process whereby play both reflects *and* contributes to the development of the child in all areas. **Table 1-1** summarizes the development of play. However, additional factors influence the expression of play across all ages. One of the most important of these is gender.

Gender Differences

Differences in gendered play have been noted in modern times as well as in children of early societies (Barnes, 2006). Male children in Greek society learned physical prowess and athletics through play. Early males played marbles and played with models of war ships and other toys meant to instill ability with hunting and fighting. Girls in early societies played with miniature pots and pans, similar to the later tea parties and toys meant for playing house. Similar gender differences in play preferences have been repeatedly studied and consistently found in a variety of more modern settings using multiple methods (Benenson, 1993; Benjamin, 1932; Caldera, Huston, & O'Brien, 1989; Connor & Serbin, 1977; Fein, 1981; Honig, 2006; Meyer-Bahlburg, Sandberg, Dolezal, & Yager, 1994; O'Brien & Huston, 1985; Pelligrini, 1992; Saracho, 1990; Servin, Bohlin, & Berlin, 1999; Wall, Pickert, & Gibson, 1989). Researchers have found that generally girls prefer toys such as dolls and house toys (like a tea set), whereas boys prefer transportation and construction toys such as blocks (Benjamin, 1932; Fein, 1981; Servin et al., 1999).

Table 1-1 Summary of the Development of Play

Age	Object Play	Motor Play	Pretend Play	Social Play
Infancy	Mostly single-object use, although combining of objects begins to emerge by the end of the first year. Uses objects in sensorimotor ways.	Reflexive or random actions become more likely to be repeated as the infant gets older and has more motor control. Early motor play includes manipulating, banging, and throwing.	Begins to emerge about age 1 year.	Visual attention and focus develops, leading to joint attention; social referencing emerges. Infant is initially more interested in objects than peers, but interest in peers increases by the end of the first year.
Toddlerhood	Increasingly combines objects and uses objects appropriately. Trial and error and invention occurs.	Exploration of greater distances and learning to walk, run, climb, and jump.	Beginning simple pretense (wave bye-bye, talk into pretend phone); most pretense is about self, and often pretense is imitative.	Social referencing increases. Increased interest in peers occurs. Toddlers do have friends and friendship is generated by imitation. Onlooker play at age 1 becomes parallel and then associative by age 3.
Preschool Years	Uses a variety of objects and enjoys combining objects. Constructive play is quite common.	Exercise play or practice play occurs. Intense gross motor activities and physical challenges often sought after.	Early preschoolers combine scenes into simple narratives. Pretend play extends to objects and others; pretense becomes more inventive, creative, and increasingly supported by language. By age 5 child can create complex scenes and direct characters and others; characters seem to act on their own. They also begin to use language to inform others of the play: "Pretend that…".	Has definite friends and enjoys play with others. Begins associative play and moves into cooperative play before kindergarten.
Elementary/ Middle Childhood	Constructs elaborate creations with a variety of materials. Leisure crafts may begin.	Engages in rough and tumble play and games with rules.	Simple pretend play declines. Engages in complex fantasy games and may begin to play specific games with pretend elements such as Dungeons and Dragons.	Seeks companions for play and processes more complex play activities with others.
Adolescence	May continue with leisure crafts/hobbies.	Greater participation in recreation and sports.	Engagement in theater, fantasy games, and video games with entire worlds online.	Teamwork and cooperation develop; begins to "hang out" with friends.

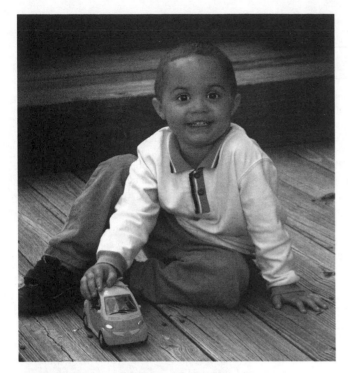

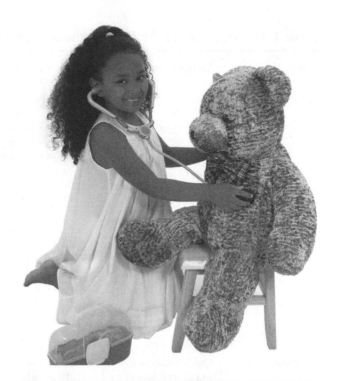

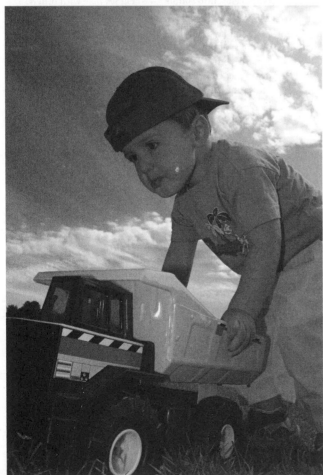

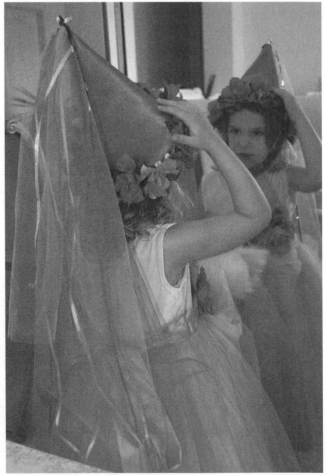

Boys often prefer transportation and construction toys.

Girls often prefer doll play and dress up.

Children often request toys that are labeled for their gender (Bradbard & Parkman, 1983; O'Brien & Huston, 1985; Martin, Eisenbud, & Rose, 1995; Servin et al., 1999). Additionally, the gender labels given to toys may affect a child's desire for that plaything (Martin et al., 1995). Amazingly, children appear to require only a rudimentary understanding of gender to learn gender stereotypes and exhibit these gender-based toy preferences (Martin & Little, 1990).

Gendered preferences can be seen at various ages. As early as 1 year of age, children make different toy choices based on gender (Servin et al., 1999). At 18 months, boys choose play with trucks, trailers, men, and logs, whereas girls choose doll-related activities (Lyytinen, Laakso, Poikkeus, & Rita, 1999). Boys are more likely to choose physical and block play over dramatic and manipulative play (Saracho, 1990). Connor and Serbin (1977) observed preschool-age children's play choices and found boys preferred blocks, balls, transportation toys, construction toys, and gross motor play. Girls in the study preferred crayons, dolls and dollhouses, musical instruments and painting, reading, sewing cards, and the play telephone.

Boys and girls not only choose different toys but also choose different playmates and ways of playing (Benenson, 1993; Hartup, 1983). At a very young age, both genders prefer same-sex groupings, and this preference continues until adolescence. Girls prefer to interact in dyads or smaller groups, with greater cooperation, whereas boys prefer larger groups and more competition. Girls are generally rated as more playful than boys and engage in more verbal pretending (Saunders, Sayer, & Goodale, 1999; Von Klitzing, Kelsay, Emde, Robinson, & Schmitz, 2000; Wall et al., 1989).

Boys are more likely to enjoy vigorous or active play, rough and tumble play, and outdoor play (Eaton & Enns, 1986; Humphreys, & Smith, 1987; Pellegrini, 1988, 1992, 1995). Boys' physical play often has a fantasy theme, such as playing super heroes (Pellegrini & Bjorklund, 2004), and boys display aggressive play more than girls (Goldstein, 1995; Power, 2000). Some believe that boys are biologically prone to a greater activity level and a preference for more active play. However, some research has suggested that both boys and girls have a similar activity level and that both exhibit a greater activity level with toys and activities stereotyped as masculine (O'Brien & Huston, 1985).

Toys that are gender stereotyped may actually alter the nature of parent–child interaction during play, regardless of the gender of the parent being observed or the gender of the child (Caldera et al., 1989). For example, in play with toys labeled as masculine (such as trucks), researchers found interaction styles that demonstrated lower levels of questioning, less teaching, and less proximity between parents and children. However, these types of toys elicited more parental sounds and more verbal corrections of behavior. Feminine toys generated interaction styles with close physical proximity and greater verbal interaction. Neutral toys, such as puzzles, generated greater positive and informative verbalizations from parents (Caldera et al., 1989).

Are these gender differences still found today? Are they real? Since the mid-1900s, gender roles have changed, and the family form has changed as well (DaVanzo & Rahman, 1993; Schor, 2003). There has also been a push toward more gender-neutral play (Barnes, 2006). One might believe that the cultural revolution, greater awareness, and the huge changes in men's and women's roles in this country could affect gendered play choices. However, gender differences continue to be found in more recent research with video games. Boys play video games more frequently and for longer periods (Kafai, 1998) and tend to play more competitive and risky games. Girls prefer games with social interactions and greater character development (Salonius-Pasternak & Gelfond, 2005). Girls appear to enjoy participating in a story more than participating in a competitive game. The body of literature on humans, along with the large research base on gender differences in animal behavior, suggests that continuing, real gender-based differences in play may be biological. These differences may be encouraged or hindered depending on cultural or contextual factors in the home and the community.

Contextual Features That Impact What Children Play or Like to Play

A variety of environmental factors could influence a child's preferences for play. Children must play with what and whom they have available to them. Therefore, affluence or poverty, and community wellness or social strife can impact development, play choices, and children's overall participation in daily occupations (De Barros, Fragosos, de Oliveira, Filho, & de Castro, 2003; Engel-Yeger, Jarus, & Law, 2007; Ginsburg, American Academy of Pediatrics Committee on Communications, & American Academy of Pediatrics Committee on Psychosocial Aspects of Child and Family Health, 2007).

Even with limited means, children find things to play with. If children are able to safely access natural landscapes, they will find much to play with. Although they have few toys, children living in hunter-gatherer societies use materials available to them to create a variety of outdoor games and playful activities (Gosso et al., 2005). There are games of balance, games in the trees, water play, spinning games using fruits, games using slingshots and bows and arrows, games building with sand and mud, and social games similar to hide and seek. These forms of play are often very enjoyable, and even children with access to commercial toys often prefer play *in* nature and *with* nature.

Children without commercial toys can also create toys from whatever materials are available (Edwards, 2005). Adult "trash" often can be used to fashion toys, and very elaborate and imaginative games can be made from buttons, bottle caps, paper, scraps of cloth, cans, and so on (Edwards, 2005). Therefore, play is often more complex when children reside in an area where there are plentiful trash materials. Many children grow up in areas and neighborhoods where what they play is hindered by the context in which they find themselves. Certain neighborhoods or areas that are unsafe, whether due to crime or to war, may reduce the amount of outdoor physical play that occurs and may also reduce access to the natural materials and trash materials with which to fashion toys (Edwards, 2005).

In stark contrast, not all children grow up with limited means, and affluence can also impact play preferences. Today some authors are concerned with the commercialization of toys for affluent children (Scarlett et al., 2005). Children from affluent homes in the United States, for example, have excessive numbers of toys available to them of multiple different types. However, the purchasing of large quantities of toys, in some cases, may be an effort to get children to "go play" alone rather than with parents or other adults (Scarlett et al., 2005). Affluent children also may be "overscheduled" with daily structured activities and may not be allowed to choose freely how to spend their play time with peers (American Occupational Therapy Association, 2008; Elkind, 2001; Ginsburg et al., 2007; Rigby & Rodger, 2006). It is not yet clear what the impact of these changes in play will be for today's children.

Another important contextual feature in the development of play preferences is one's peers. Peer cultures develop through play via shared meanings regarding the use of objects and spaces and shared themes of play (Elgas, Klein, Kantor, & Fernie, 1988; Kantor, Elgas, & Fernie, 1993). Certain objects can be used by young children in specific ways to gain access to peer group membership. These peer-specific forms of play can be quite pervasive within one peer group but nonexistent in other peer groups. Although peer cultures can be quite individual from place to place, the increasing usage of media (television, movies, and video games) by young children has increased the possibility of shared play themes among peers at varying locations across communities—even across the entire United States. A child who has seen the movie *Cars* in New York can pretend play the movie theme with cousins in Nebraska.

Therefore, media could be considered an additional contextual feature that may influence play preferences. Not only does media influence peer cultures in children, but some believe the explosion of media in the last century may have actually altered the way in which children play (Singer & Singer, 2005). As noted previously, children spend more time in sedentary play (Clements, 2004; Singer & Singer, 2001) often in front of video games,

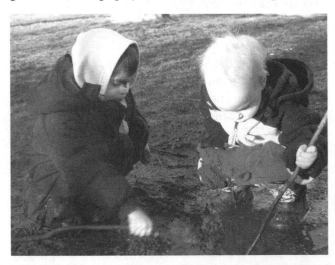

Nature provides many opportunities for play without the need for commerical toys.

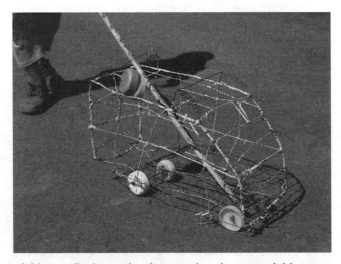

Children will play with whatever they have available, even building toys from adult "trash."

television, movies, or computer games. Outdoor play has also diminished dramatically (Rivkin, 2006). Overall, the impact of media on children may be difficult to quantify, but it has not gone unnoticed by marketing companies.

In this country at least, a large part of advertising is targeted at children specifically to influence their play choices. According to the National Institute on Media and the Family[5] (Strasburger, 2001), a typical child in America may see as many as 40,00 television ads per year. For all forms of media, advertisers may spend almost $12 billion a year targeting children. Studies of the effects of advertising on children suggest that ads do influence the choices and preferences of children in terms of toys and other goods (Gunter & Furnham, 1998). The extent of media influences on children's play preferences is unclear as of yet.

What Do Children with Disabilities Play?

As occupational therapists, we must be informed not only about the play of typically developing children but also about the play of children with disabilities. There is little literature on the play of children with disabilities compared with the enormous body of work on typical play development. However, we know that although children with disabilities do play and appear to have similar playful attitudes to non-disabled peers, they play differently from children without disabilities (Ferland, 2005).

Children with disabilities often progress through similar stages of play development as children without disabilities but at delayed ages and reduced rates (Gowen et al., 1992). Children with physical limitations deal with barriers to accessing free play and limited free choice of activities (Missiuna & Pollack, 1991; Pollack et al., 1997). They need greater assistance to play from adults in their environment (Skar, 2002). Research has shown that children with physical disabilities spend more time in passive activities (Brown & Gordon, 1987), demonstrate less active involvement with objects (Gowen et al., 1992), and spend more time with adults rather than peers, participating in activities such as television watching rather than active and varied play experiences (Howard, 1996).

Children with mild motor impairments may still have poor play skills (Bundy, 1989; Clifford & Bundy, 1989). Children with learning disabilities but minimal physical limitations play alone more often than their peers without learning disabilities (Gottlieb, Gottlieb, Berkell, & Levy, 1986). Children with visual impairments spend less

time in play with peers, spend more time with adults, and often engage in perseverative or stereotypical play (Skellenger, Rosenblum, & Jager, 1997). The difficulties in the play of children with autism are well documented (Rogers, Cook, & Meryl, 2005) and include lack of symbolic play, less motivation to play, limited imitation of others in play, and repetitive play with objects.

Play choices may be more related to developmental age than chronological age. Because the development of play behaviors is closely tied to cognitive and motor development, the development of play in children with disabilities, therefore may be less affected by changes in chronological age. Often, for children with severe disabilities, skills improve slowly. When play was observed over a 3-year period in a sample of children with disabilities, little change was found in play behaviors (Sigafoos, Roberts-Pennell, & Graves, 1999). Interestingly, when studying the play behavior of children with intellectual disability, Messier, Ferland, and Majnemer (2008) found no relationship between IQ level and individual dimensions of the play assessment, the Assessment of Ludic Behavior. These authors did find that motor play was a strength for this population. Additionally, these children were curious, took initiative in play, demonstrated enjoyment, and sought out sensory-based play. These children were less likely to demonstrate high scores on sense of humor and enjoyment of challenge.

Playfulness has been studied in children with various disabilities with varying results. Children with sensory integrative dysfunction exhibited less playful play than typically developing peers (Bundy, 1989). A case study of a child with sensory processing issues demonstrated that this child had very cautious and repetitive play with limited familiar choices (Benson, Nicka, & Stern, 2006). Another study of children with developmental disabilities also found differences in playfulness between these children and control children who were typically developing (Hamm, 2006). In a variety of studies, Bundy and colleagues demonstrated limited playfulness in children with autism (Muys, Rodger, & Bundy, 2006; Reed, Dunbar, & Bundy, 2000; Skaines, Rodger, & Bundy, 2006) and other disabilities (Leipold & Bundy, 2000). Similarly, children with cerebral palsy demonstrated less playful play than their typically developing peers (Okimoto, Bundy, & Hanzlik, 2000). However, one study (Harkness & Bundy, 2001) found no differences between those with and without physical disabilities in terms of playfulness. The authors thought perhaps this was due to high scores of exuberance in the children with physical disabilities or due to measurement in familiar environments.

---

[5] see *http://www.mediafamily.org/index.shtml*

Differences in play skills or the ability to access play do not necessarily equate to differences in play preferences. Although one can readily observe actual play *behaviors*, examining the play *preferences* of children with disabilities is more difficult because physical limitations may hinder access to preferred activities, and limited communication may hinder discussion. It can be difficult, therefore, to determine the true preferences of some children with disabilities, and this may be the reason we currently know so little about the preferences of children with both physical and cognitive impairments.

Research is just beginning to examine the play preferences of children with disabilities. Thus far, the studies have demonstrated, not surprisingly, that children with disabilities can and do indicate specific play preferences. For example, children with an autism spectrum disorder have been found to demonstrate clear preferences for play activities and objects with sensorimotor properties, favored characters, and predictable situations (Desha, Ziviani, & Roger, 2003; Ferrara & Hill, 1980). Children with developmental delays are reported by their parents to exhibit a preference for rough and tumble play and gross motor play above more sedentary play such as watching television, drawing, or coloring (Case-Smith & Miller Kuhaneck, 2008). Children with physical disabilities who were asked about their play choices and the technical aids they needed for play indicated they enjoyed play and thought play was fun, and many played typical games for their age and gender. However, many reported barriers to outdoor play because of poor physical access to play environments (Skar, 2002). Therefore, many of these children reported they preferred indoor play and passive activities, which is different from preferred activities reported by typically developing children.

So do children with disabilities have different preferences from typically developing children? One study found that children with mild motor disabilities hold preferences similar to children without disabilities (Clifford & Bundy, 1989), whereas another study (Case-Smith & Miller Kuhaneck, 2008) found differences in preferences. In a recent survey of parents of children with and without disabilities, the play preferences of children aged 3 to 7 were examined and compared (Case-Smith & Miller Kuhaneck, 2008). From a sample of 83 children with developmental delay and a total sample of 166 children, the authors found no gender differences in play preferences within this age group but did find expected age-related changes. In addition, the preferences of the typical and developmentally delayed children were somewhat different. Children with

developmental delays preferred rough and tumble play more than typically developing children, and typically developing children preferred quiet table-top activities more than the children with developmental delays. Additionally, typically developing children reportedly preferred play with peers more than children with developmental delays (Case-Smith & Miller Kuhaneck, 2008).

Although we do not know for sure, and the research is limited to date, it is likely that children with disabilities at similar developmental levels as their non-disabled peers hold play preferences similar to their peers. Their preferences may be shaped by physical or cognitive limitations that restrict their access to certain play opportunities, however. A more thorough examination of the impact of cognitive and physical disabilities on play preferences is warranted because it has practical implications for activity choices in therapeutic interventions.

Question: What do children like to play?

Answer: Children create individual play preferences. Different children like to play different things and these choices are based on a variety of factors both within and outside of the child. The factors that impact choices include gender, age and the related cognitive and motor skill development that comes with age, and cultural and contextual features of the child's environment and surroundings. At different points in a child's life, different factors may become more prominent or recede in importance, but in the end, every individual grows up with a combination of childhood play experiences and preferences that is unique to that individual.

■ WHERE DOES PLAY OCCUR?

Play happens all over the world and has been observed in many cultures and within many forms of societal structure (Edwards, 2005; Gosso et al., 2005; Lancy, 1996; Nwokah & Ikekeonwu, 1998). Western industrialized cultures have increasingly afforded more importance to play. Children in these cultures are therefore often provided with specific places for play such as playgrounds, playrooms, and commercial play areas. Some of these can be quite elaborate.

There is significant variation across the globe, however, in the places where play occurs. Elaborate playgrounds, woods with trees to climb, or streams and rivers to swim in are not evenly distributed. In very rural locations across the globe, play, by necessity, occurs in fields,

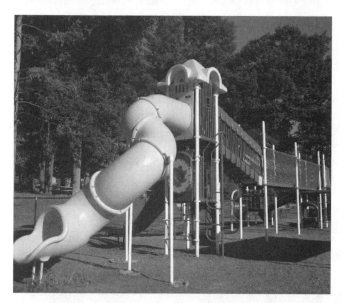

In some cultures, children are provided elaborate places to play.

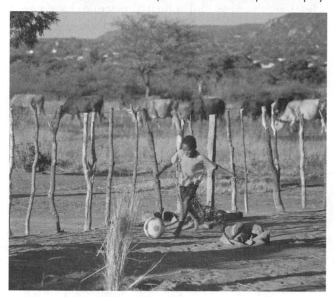

Play will happen in the spaces that are available.

in the dirt or grassy spaces between homes, in the local woods, or in the home (Lancy, 1996; Nwokah & Ikekeonwu, 1998).

Features of environments, the "where" of play, likely impact play behaviors. One study comparing the games of Nigerian children and American children found that the overall participation in categories of play was similar between the cultures. However, the terrain where the children's games were played was different, thus somewhat altering the specific games available to the children (Nwokah & Ikekeonwu, 1998).

Another issue to consider in terms of where play occurs is whether it happens near adults or away from adults.

In certain cultures, play is more likely to occur with or without adults nearby (Edwards, 2005; Lancy, 1996; Nwokah & Ikekeonwu, 1998). For example, in many hunter-gatherer societies, children under age 7 are encouraged to play together, away from adults, to allow adults to work (Gosso et al., 2005). In many farming and industrial societies, boys in middle childhood in particular roam away from home in gender-segregated groups to play (Edwards, 2005). In other cultures, children are encouraged to stay near adults, observe adults, and participate in the "work" of the community. As a result, play happens near the adults during or in between work chores (Bazyk, Stalnaker, Llerena, Ekelman, & Bazyk, 2003; Lancy, 1996).

> **Question:** Where does play occur?
>
> **Answer:** Anywhere it can. Children will play anywhere they are able, but the structure and content of their play may differ based on the play spaces they have available to them.

■ WHEN DOES PLAY OCCUR?

Play can occur almost anytime. One prerequisite for play to occur, however, is a feeling of safety and security. In both humans and nonhuman species, play occurs when basic survival needs are met and there is at least a minimum level of safety. Play is often the first activity to be lost, however, when things are not going well for an animal (Bateson, 2005).

Whenever a child is not otherwise occupied, for example, with school or chores, the child can play. In addition, children can approach those work tasks with a playful attitude (Glynn, 1994) and play while they are working (Bazyk et al., 2003; Lancy, 1996; Nwokah & Ikekeonwu, 1998).

There has tended to be an artificially created division by many play researchers that identified two different constructs: work and play. These two terms were often considered to be mutually exclusive, ignoring the idea that one could play while working or that one could take one's play very seriously and approach it almost like work (Holmes, 1999). There is likely a continuum between work and play rather than separate categories. Children asked to classify activities as either work or play label some things as "in between" (Wing, 1995), and this idea of a continuum has been noted in other similar studies (Holmes, 1999).

However, 5-year-olds consider the terms mutually exclusive, whereas college students do not, suggesting that an understanding of the continuum may require a certain cognitive level or level of experience (Holmes, 1999).

One other distinction needs to be made in terms of the "when" of play. As stated earlier in the chapter, some researchers divide play into two types: exploration and true play. These authors suggest that for play to occur, the play object must be fully explored. The child must know the characteristics of the object to know what the object can do (Hutt, 1966). We disagree with this. For our purposes, exploration is often an aspect of play, and we believe an appropriate level of novelty and exploration is necessary for play to continue. Simple objects can become rapidly boring if they are unable to be used in multiple ways. Children stop playing, as do some animals, when the play object lacks novelty. In a study of cats, habituation to a cat toy led to the stoppage of play, whereas reintroduction of novelty led to the return of play (Hall, 1998). Novelty was important to the maintenance of play behavior over time. As therapists, we have all seen the child who becomes bored with a game or object without any flexibility. Therefore, exploration is not a prerequisite for when play occurs, but rather exploration can also occur during play.

> **Question:** When do children play?
>
> **Answer:** They play whenever they can. They will play when they feel safe and when they are not required to do something else (and even sometimes when they are required to do something else). They will play when they are alone or with others. They will play at any point of the day and will even sometimes play long past the need for sleep. The "when" of play is almost anytime as long as children are safe and their survival needs are met.

■ WHY DO CHILDREN PLAY?

There are many possible functions of play. Play may allow children to work out psychological issues and difficulties they are dealing with in the present. Play may help children prepare for adult roles and responsibilities. Play may help youngsters develop motor skills and promote cognitive and social development (Ginsburg et al., 2007). In this way, play can be considered as "developmental scaffolding" (Bateson, 2005, p. 16). These different statements regarding the functions of play indicate broad traditions of theories regarding the purpose of play.

Early Theories of the Function of Play

In this section, early theories of the function of play are highlighted briefly. Much of this work has been explored extensively elsewhere, and because these theories are not the focus of this text, interested readers are encouraged to seek out the original authors as cited or other summaries of their work for more in-depth consideration.

Play to Burn Off or to Restore Energy

One of the earliest theories of play, the surplus energy theory, is associated with the works of a German poet named Schiller (1875) and of Herbert Spencer (1873). They contended that play emerged in individuals and animals that had more energy than they needed for basic survival and therefore, played to "blow off steam." Although there may be some apparent logic in this, because often children seem to need to run and play when they have been sitting in school, for example, and animals do seem to have a need to romp and frolic after being confined, there are many critics of this theory, and over time it has been seen to be too limited in scope. Children do play when they are at the brink of exhaustion, and some play actually seems to refresh or rejuvenate the individual. Others believed that play served a restorative function; individuals played to refresh themselves, and, particularly with sedentary city life, people needed to use their muscles and engage in activities in more natural outdoor environments. These theories, however, cannot explain play that is more cognitive in nature, such as puzzle play. Additionally, they cannot account for play that is scary, stressful, or highly competitive and not at all relaxing (Saracho & Spodek, 1998).

Play as Preparation Versus Play as Legacy from the Past

Two other early theories proposed conflicting temporal conceptualizations of play (Burghardt, 1998): first, play was considered to be preparation for the future, and second, play was a legacy from the past. A Swiss scientist named Karl Groos (1901) proposed play as an instinct or programmed response and suggested that play was important to prepare animals and children for the skills and abilities they would need in adult life. Aspects of this theory have been carried forward into more modern theories of play, but as Groos proposed it, the theory is too limited to explain all aspects of play. However, it is true that animals with more complex adult lives tend to have longer periods of childhood and more complex ways of playing.

G. Stanley Hall's recapitulation theory, based on the ideas of Darwin, suggested that the play of each generation instinctively repeated the work of prior generations in a developmental sequence (Pellegrini & Smith, 2005; Saracho & Spodek, 1998). Children's play repeats the history of *Homo sapiens:* first come the survival pursuits of the animal, then the experiences of the early human nomadic peoples, and then agricultural and tribal stages. The young boy climbing a tree is expressing his primate past, whereas the older child play fighting is expressing his or her hunter-gatherer past. This theory has been discounted for multiple reasons, and there are many forms of play that hold little relationship to any past human history (e.g., hang gliding or video games). However, Hall's work did stimulate later study of the developmental stages of play, and for that, it is important. In addition, Hall promoted the importance of play in childhood and believed that play and exploration should be allowed and supported.

Play to Develop Cognition

The cognitive developmental tradition of child development suggests that play allows children to develop and integrate new skills and abilities into their repertoire. Cognitive theorists in this tradition include Piaget (1952/1975), Vygotsky (1976), and Bruner (1982). Piaget provided detailed descriptions of cognitive development noted through his children's play. Vygotsky, initially working on language and child development, introduced the notion of a "zone of proximal development." This zone is the area where a child is stretched to a slightly higher level of functioning but one that is not outside the realm of his or her capabilities. This stretching occurs with the help of another individual of higher skill. Bruner's major contribution is in the idea of scaffolding, which is the support of another person. Each of these cognitive theories has been used to explain play.

Play can develop and expand because adults and more skilled peers help children to participate in higher levels of play than children would participate in alone. As a group, these cognitive theorists believed that play expressed or reflected children's learning and that children learned through play. Although play indicates cognitive and motor development and may assist development, it may not be absolutely necessary for development. For example, children from non-Western cultures where play is not encouraged or promoted still develop and learn (Bazyk et al., 2003; Gosso et al., 2005).

Play to Develop Emotional Well-Being

Another view of play is promoted by psychoanalysts such as Freud and Erickson (1950). In the views of this tradition, the function of play is to allow children to make sense of their feelings. Play allows children to reduce their feelings of helplessness. Play allows children to gain a sense of control over situations, to work through loss or grief, and to deal with anger in an acceptable fashion. There are many critics of these theories[6] because they do ignore the many other types of play in much younger children and in animals that lack the wide range of emotions experienced by humans. This theory also cannot explain a wide variety of recreational activities such as collecting and hiking.

Play to Be Engaged

Other researchers, including Berlyne (1960), described play as an intrinsically motivated activity that arises because of the need to seek arousal when one is not adequately stimulated by the environment. The focus of these theories is on the innate curiosity for exploration that is often seen in play and the "fun" of assimilating novel information. Some focus on play as an escape from boredom. Others focus on the sensory aspects of activities, believing that individuals choose activities based on the sensory experiences they provide and that those choices reflect an individual's need for sensation (Zuckerman, 1971). White (1959) proposed a theory of motivation that explains play as a persistent urge to interact effectively with the environment. Children gain competence through play and thus adapt and grow into functional adults. Satisfaction is gained through competent interactions with the environment, and children gain pleasure from the ability to do something. Although the theory states that play allows competence to build in children who play, the goal of the children who are playing is not to build competence—it is to have fun. As a whole, the theories in this group appear logical but cannot account for the entire range of motivation to play, nor for the continuum of playful work and "workful" play.

Current Biological Theories

Many of the newer theories of play have emerged from the study of the play of animals within the field of evolutionary biology. It is important to consider why other species play because there is likely to be an advantage to this behavior for it to continue. One must also consider that in many species, play is quite costly (Bateson, 2005; Bekoff & Byers, 1998). There is an expenditure of energy and the potential of being viewed and attacked by predators,

---

[6] see *http://www.psychotherapy.ro/resources/uncategorized/psychoanalysis-criticisms/*

and play in some species can be dangerous, such as when seal pups are killed by sea lions while they play. Play also seems to disappear when animals are under stress, suggesting that it is in fact costly to the animal to engage in it (Burghardt, 1984). So, what advantage could play provide for a species? Why does it continue throughout long periods of human and animal evolution?

Play to Prepare for Adulthood

One popular theory is that play in juvenile animals prepares the animal for adulthood (Bateson, 2005; Bekoff, 2002; Fry, 2005; Thompson, 1998). Support of this theory is that play behaviors in animals are often noted to be facsimiles of risky adult behaviors such as catching prey, avoiding predation, fighting, and mating. Generally, play forms do not exist for nonrisky behaviors, such as grooming or urinating. So perhaps play evolved because it enabled practice of potentially dangerous adult behaviors during childhood. Although this "preparation for adulthood" theory seems logical, evidence often contradicts it. The movements used in animal play in childhood are often different from those used in adulthood. And during play fighting, as opposed to real fighting, when things get too rough, one animal will back down or ease off to allow play to continue (Bekoff, 2002; Fry, 2005; Thompson, 1998). This does not occur in real violent contests. Some aspects of play fighting are actually counterproductive to learning real fighting (Biben, 1998). For example, in squirrel monkeys, mismatched play partners go out of their way to make partners feel safe. They play fair or they do not play. There is also little evidence that animals that do play at something in their youth are better at it in adulthood (Caro, 1994).

Another theory of play in animals suggests that play provides exercise to the motor skills that are necessary in adulthood. However, there is much evidence to contradict this theory (Byers, 1998; Thompson, 1998). For example, during play, the motions used are often too short in duration to provide any real muscular benefit. If play is for exercise, why are some play bouts in animals so brief? Generally, play bouts are not enough for exercise in terms of muscular changes. Also, if play is for muscular exercise, why does it not begin right at birth and continue throughout life? Instead, play peaks in the juvenile period, but muscular development declines rapidly if exercise is not continued. If play is for the muscular development of children, there should be evidence that play increases the survival of children; however, there is no evidence of this. The evidence contradicting the idea that the purpose of play is preparation for adult activities has

led animal researchers to propose other rationales (Byers, 1998; Thompson, 1998).

Play to Build Social Competence

One alternative rationale for play in animals may be greater learning of the local environment, the members of the social group, and the local culture. Bekoff (2002) suggested that perhaps play allows animals to learn fairness and social morality. So, perhaps social play therefore serves the function of acquisition of social competence. Researchers studying the effects of play deprivation in rats found that lack of play during specific periods can influence later social behavior (Hol, Van den Berg, Van Ree, & Spruijt, 1999; Van den Berg et al., 1999). Isolated animals fail to learn playfulness and social play and often react to other animals with aggressive or fearful behaviors (Lewis, 2005). So, perhaps play promotes socialization. Similarly, Panksepp and colleagues (Panksepp & Burgdorf, 2003; Panksepp, Burgdorf, Turner, & Gordon, 2003) studied the social emotional implications of play including a behavior in rats that they consider laughter. Their research suggests that play serves important social functions in rat development.

Play as a Test of Competence

Thompson (1998) suggested that perhaps play is a mechanism of managing development so as to provide feedback on one's abilities in relation to others, in an effort to regulate future activities. Play choices allow one to examine one's own competence level. An observation supporting this theory is that the outcome of play is often success or failure, winning or losing. Juveniles do choose activities that are at the right level of challenge, not too easy or too

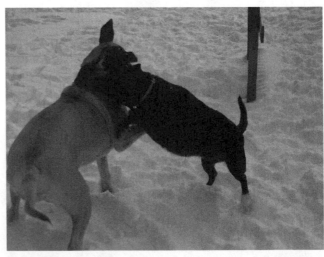

Does play fighting occur in preparation of the real thing? Not according to some research.

hard. They will "change the test" if it is too easy and will continue until they fail the test. They also need novelty and greater challenge in their play, creating new tests as their abilities improve. Thompson (1998) suggested that these play tests and the search for novelty was favored by evolution, because those who were most able to assess their competence in a full range of activities before needing the skills for survival were more likely to survive.

Play to Promote Creativity and Flexibility

Play's greatest benefit may be the ability of an individual to modify behavior creatively and flexibly in the face of changes in conditions. Play may enhance creativity and the facilitation of innovation and problem solving (Bateson, 2005). There would be an evolutionary advantage for those creatures that played and that were able to respond more adaptively to novel situations. This may not have been the original purpose of the development of play on the planet but a fortunate by-product (Bateson, 2005). Many theorists have begun to consider the idea that a strong benefit of play that may have led to continued evolution is that play creates more flexible brains that are able to respond creatively to novel problems.

Play to Create Neurological Flexibility

A currently popular theory suggests that the one feature common to all forms of play in all species is that play promotes flexible brains (Sutton-Smith, 1997). Play leads to a broader mental repertoire that helps an animal be successful in adult life, whether in the areas of social interactions, obtaining food, or avoiding predation. During play, random actions are common. Play creates the unexpected and allows animals to learn to deal with novelty (Spinka, Newberry, & Bekoff, 2001).

Sutton-Smith (1997) discussed that the most common concept among all various writings on play is variability, and perhaps variability is what play is all about. He suggested that play assists in the actualization of brain potential, in saving of more brain variability, and perhaps in creating novel brain connections to enhance the child's potential variability. Play helps us face our fears and see possibilities, and helps us be optimistic and creative (Sutton-Smith, 1997). In terms of evolution, the function of play is to enhance survival by allowing for more flexible and variable solutions to the typical problems of everyday existence. He therefore defined play as "a facsimilization of the struggle for survival as this is broadly rendered by Darwin" (Sutton-Smith, 1997, p. 231). If the purpose of play is to promote brain growth, development, and flexibility,

then there should be indications of this in brain research. New methods of investigating the brain's structures and functions support these new theories.

Studies of the play behaviors of rats and the brain mechanisms for play have supported the new theories on the role of play in flexibility and brain development. Scientists are beginning to examine the specific functions of brain structures and regions in play. Play has been specifically linked to the development of the cerebellum (Byers, 1998). In both rats and cats, the growth curves of the cerebellum match the growth and decline of play rates in these species. Play occurs and peaks at ages when it is possible for motor activity to alter the formation of synapses in the brain areas responsible for motor control. Cerebellar synapse formation can be influenced by the environment; experience mediates which synapses are retained and the number of synapses per cell. These effects appear to be permanent, so that when the development of the cerebellum is completed, play stops (or slows).

Other brain areas are involved as well. Rough and tumble play in particular activates many areas of the brain, and the pinning behaviors of rats appears to be related to the parafascicular region of the thalamus, an area that may be responsible for integration of somatosensory information during play (Siviy, 1998). The amygdala and the dorsolateral frontal cortex have been shown to be related to play as well. In rats who were allowed to play for 30 minutes, these areas had significantly elevated brain-derived neurotrophic factor mRNA expression (Gordon, Burke, Akil, Watson, & Panksepp, 2003). The motor cortex may be required to allow for the alteration of play patterns to environmental contexts (Kamitakahara, Monfils, Forgie, Kolb, & Pellis, 2007). Specifically, damage to the orbitofrontal cortex in early life may alter the ability to modify patterns of response in play fighting with different patterns (Pellis et al., 2006). With the widespread neurological impact of play, play could facilitate a brain with a greater number of response options and could facilitate coping, creativity, and learning, thereby supporting the previously mentioned theories of "play as flexibility."

The neurotransmitters of dopamine, norepinephrine, and serotonin have all been found to play a role in play behaviors (Siviy, 1998). Dopamine is important for the increased arousal needed before a play bout and the anticipatory behaviors before play, whereas norepinephrine and serotonin modulate capacity for play once the animal is playing. Animals with low norepinephrine play less, whereas those with low serotonin play more. Low serotonin may increase play by altering the animal's responsiveness to playful overtures of others. These neurotransmitters also have widespread impact throughout the brain.

Perhaps play *is* a mechanism of promoting brain development. Would this mean that animals that play more would have larger brains? In primates, social play is correlated with brain size. Larger social groups create a greater cognitive load, and therefore, greater brain size may have evolved in species living in larger social groupings. However, research evidence does not completely support this assumption (Iwaniuk, Nelson, & Pellis, 2001). More likely is that play is related to size of specific brain areas or structures that are highly related to play (Pellis & Iwaniuk, 2002).

If play is for promoting brain development, the absence of play should be visible in the brain as well. There is now some emerging evidence in rats of neurological effects of play deprivation (Henig, 2008). Pellis and colleagues are also currently studying the neurological impact of play deprivation[7] for current research projects. In these studies of play-deprived rats, there is an immature pattern of neural connections, where appropriate neural pruning seems to have been missed or skipped. However, this is an area of study in its infancy.

A New Way to Consider Why Children Play

Much confusion exists in the research and writing about why children play. Some researchers have therefore begun to consider that perhaps while searching for the purpose of play, they have been studying aspects of play that are not play's primary evolutionary purpose but instead just beneficial consequences. One author argued that scientists must separate the *cause* of play from the *function* of play (Burghardt, 1984, 2005). Examining the function of play may not lead any closer to the evolutionary *cause* of play. One needs to consider the primary processes that led to play evolving in ancient animals separately from the secondary processes, which have evolved over time as play conferred additional evolutionary benefits on animals that engaged in it.

Perhaps certain situations had to occur before play could evolve (Burghardt, 1984, 2005). Certain species may have been physiologically more or less adapted to originate play. For example, reptiles have curiosity, arousal, learning mechanisms, and exploration, but they do not demonstrate play as people usually think of it. Reptiles rely on external heat; they have anaerobic metabolism and little parental care. These conditions make play an inappropriate strategy for reptiles. Perhaps early species to originate play were more efficient in their use of their metabolic energy. Perhaps play initially evolved in those species with a set growth rate and excess energy. Play appears to occur in species with protected childhoods and parental care, the capacity for rapid learning, and the need for quick movements and flexibility. Burghardt (1984) suggested that play emerged initially out of exploration to escape boredom in animals where food was plentiful, where predators perhaps were limited, and where parental care provided for most needs. After a period of evolution where length of parental care increased, play evolved to facilitate rapid behavioral and mental development through natural selection. Through mechanisms of evolution, play continued because of a host of secondary and tertiary benefits (**Figure 1-4**) (Burghardt, 1984, 2005).

Figure 1-4   Process of Play

Primary Processes

- Sufficient metabolic energy
- Animals buffered from severe stress and food shortages
- High activity levels or the need for stimulation to elicit typical behavior systems and optimal arousal
- Complex behaviors in varying conditions

Secondary Processes

- Neurological benefits
- Behavioral flexibility
- Improved perceptual motor coordination
- Physical fitness

Tertiary Processes

- Improved social status and reproductive success
- Resources for novel behavior and creativity
- Ability for mental play
- Neurobehavioral development
- Reorganized and more complex behavioral systems

Adapted from Burghardt (1984, 2005)

[7] see *http://ccbn.uleth.ca/people/primary/pellis.php* and *http://www.excellence-earlychildhood.ca/repimpCopernic.asp?lang=EN&pos=348*

In considering play in this way, the multitude of apparent functions of play can be collapsed. Many of the prior theories discussed can be placed within this framework. The early theories of Groos (1901) and Spencer (1873) presented earlier in this chapter can be reconsidered in light of this model, as can the newer theories of brain flexibility, self-assessment, and social engagement. Play arose from instinctual behaviors and neural organization that provided pleasure from these motor behaviors. Play was initially rewarding and was incorporated into many behavioral systems over time. Play became adaptive in different ways in different species. Species with needs to navigate in complex environments or escape from predators have highly evolved locomotor play forms. Species that are carnivores, omnivores, and scavengers often exhibit object play. Social play is common in species that are social animals. Most likely, children play now for many reasons, not one.

Summary of Why Children Play

Although these theories too may eventually be replaced, the newer theories proposed by animal scientists that consider the influences of biology and neurology seem to come closest to explaining why children play. Children play because at some point in early history, certain necessary conditions were met. Then, a variety of beneficial consequences evolved through play that promoted survival and further evolution. Throughout time, play has served as a function to allow species that live in complex environments to thrive. Play encourages flexible thinking, creativity, and problem solving. The social aspects of play promote social-emotional bonds between individuals, and the pleasurable aspect of play promotes quality of life and mental well-being.

■ CONCLUSION

Although play seems a relatively simple phenomenon when observed, play is an incredibly complex topic to study, define, and describe. In this chapter, we provided an overview of what we believe are the important concepts relevant to play that readers need to know before continuing to the following chapters on application to intervention. General knowledge about play provides a foundation for assessing and incorporating play in occupational therapy. Interested readers are highly encouraged to seek out and read the original works cited in this chapter. The readings on the evolution of play in animals are particularly fascinating and enlightening. The study of play has finally come into its own, and the multitude of animal and cross-cultural studies being published suggest that there will be interesting new information to incorporate into theoretical frameworks in the years to come. With this introduction to the many facets of play examined by researchers in animal biology, evolutionary science, education, psychology, and child development, we next turn to the way play is viewed and used in occupational therapy.

Appendix 1-1

Web Resources on Play

PLAY

http://nifplay.org/
http://www.ipausa.org/
http://www.strongmuseum.org/
http://www.strongmuseum.org/about_play/play_journal.html
http://www.strongmuseum.org/about_play/recess_play.html
http://www.aap.org/pressroom/playFINAL.pdf
http://www.npr.org/templates/story/story.php?storyId
    =19212514
http://naecs.crc.uiuc.edu/position/recessplay.html

RIGHTS OF CHILDREN TO PLAY

http://www.righttoplay.com/site/PageServer?pagename
    =aboutRTP
http://www.playireland.ie/
http://www.ipacanada.org/home_childs.htm
http://www.unicef.org.au/SchoolRoom-Subs.asp?
    SchoolRoomID=1

PLAY IN REFUGEE CAMPS

http://www.tornfromhome.com/
http://www.savethechildren.org/publications/technical-re-
    sources/emergencies-protection/psychsocwellbeing2.pdf
http://www.refugeesinternational.org/who-we-are/our-issues

PLAY RESEARCH IN ANIMALS

http://query.nytimes.com/gst/fullpage.html?res=9404E7DA
    1339F934A25751C0A96E9C8B63&sec=&spon
    =&partner=permalink&exprod=permalink
    &pagewanted=5
http://ccbn.uleth.ca/people/primary/pellis.php
http://www-personal.umich.edu/~bclee/laughpapers.txt
http://www.youtube.com/watch?v=j-admRGFVNM
http://www.psych.umn.edu/courses/fall06/macdonalda/
    psy4960/Readings/PankseppRatLaugh_P&B03.pdf

2

Play and Pediatric Occupational Therapy: Past and Future

After reading this chapter the reader will

1. Describe the profession's views on play both historically and currently.

2. Differentiate play as an occupation from play as a skill.

3. Demonstrate an understanding of the meaning of play for children.

Deep meaning lies often in childish play.
—Johann Friedrich von Schiller

As demonstrated in Chapter One, authors in many fields of study have written about play, trying to understand why play occurs in humans and other species. Similarly, occupational therapists have been interested in and have written about play for over 40 years. As a profession, occupational therapy's thoughts on play have shifted over time, and thus the writings reflect the times in which they were written. This chapter provides an overview of play as it has been dealt with in the profession of occupational therapy, and we highlight the contributions of occupational therapy to the body of literature on play.

Currently, occupational therapy literature on play stresses the importance of examining play *as an occupation* (Bundy, 1992, 1993; Couch, Deitz, & Kanny, 1998, Knox, 1997; Parham, 2008). How does a consideration of play as an occupation differ from the way play has been discussed in prior occupational therapy literature or in literature from other fields? Before any further discussion of the distinct use of play in occupational therapy,

we must clearly define "occupation" and delineate our use of terminology.

Occupational therapists promote health, wellness, and quality of life by enabling individuals and families to engage in meaningful and preferred human occupations. There has been lengthy debate in the occupational therapy literature regarding the use of the words "occupation" and "activity." For some, the words are synonymous and used interchangeably (Fidler & Velde, 1999). However, many occupational therapy leaders have called for a clear differentiation of these terms and have attempted to provide such definitions (American Occupational Therapy Association [AOTA], 1993; Hinojosa & Blount, 2004; Nelson, 1996). In this text, we use the following definition of "occupation":

> Activities of every day life, named, organized, and given value and meaning by individuals and a culture. Occupation is everything people do to occupy themselves, including looking after themselves...enjoying life...and contributing to the social and economic fabric of their communities. (Law, Polatajko, Baptiste, & Townsend, 1997, p. 32)

In this definition and others, occupations are activities with meaning for the individual. Therefore, the same activity—for example, gardening—could be an occupation to some but not all individuals. To someone who finds gardening meaningful, it is an occupation, but to someone who does not, gardening is an activity. One person's occupation may be another person's chore. Thus the words "occupation" and "activity" are not synonymous in our usage.

The current version of the Occupational Therapy Practice Framework (AOTA, 2008) provides a variety of additional definitions for the term "occupation" gathered from leaders within the profession. Each suggests features of the core concepts of occupation. Just as the list of characteristics of play described in Chapter One helps to create a common definition of play, this listing of core concepts helps generate a shared understanding of what is meant by occupation (**Figure 2-1**). In this chapter, we will examine play as an "activity with meaning." However, we begin first with a look back to consider how our views of play in occupational therapy have changed with the times and to evaluate our contributions as a profession to the larger body of work on play.

■ OUR ROOTS IN PLAY

Although our profession is rooted firmly in our early work with adults with mental and physical disabilities, pediatric practice and play in particular have been a part of our profession since its beginnings (Meyer, 1922). The mental hygiene movement, begun initially with adults, expanded to include children with a variety of conditions throughout the early 1900s (Stevenson, 1940) as psychologists learned more about the mental difficulties of children. The field of pediatrics is a late-comer to the medical and psychological scene, however. The American Academy of Pediatrics was not established until 1930, and the American Board of Pediatrics was not established until 1933 (Luecke, 2004). The field of pediatric psychology did not

Figure 2-1   Core Concepts of Occupations

- Goal directed

- Extend over time

- May involve multiple tasks

- Have meaning to the individual participating in them

- Reflect cultural or family values

- Meet human needs

- Involve both mental and/or physical skills and abilities but may or may not have an observable physical component

- Activities that can be named in the culture

Adapted from AOTA, 2008

fully emerge as an independent discipline until the mid-1900s (Roberts, Mitchell, & McNeal, 2003). However, as mental health professionals and medical professionals became more interested in the diseases and disabilities of children, occupational therapists followed suit.

Although there is little literature in occupational therapy in the early 1900s that is specific to pediatrics, the connection between occupational therapy and the mental hygiene movement implies that children were important from the beginning of occupational therapy. One early connection between the mental hygiene movement and occupational therapy was through Hull House, a settlement house in Chicago. Members of Hull House were involved in many of the early development activities of occupational therapy (Reed & Sanderson, 1999). Jane Adams, founder of Hull House, was an influential woman in the mental hygiene movement and someone who also influenced early occupational therapists. It is clear that the individuals involved with the mental hygiene movement and the founding of occupational therapy thought children were important (Richmond, 1995). Additionally, they thought play was important. One of the first playgrounds in America was established at Hull House.[1] Julia Lathrop, a woman who lived at Hull House, taught courses in the use of crafts with patients. The courses taught by Lathrop also included play in the coursework (Dunton, 1954). One of Lathrop's students was Eleanor Clarke Slagle, one of occupational therapy's founding mothers (Reed & Sanderson, 1999).

In the middle of the 20th century, on the heels of the emergence of the field of pediatrics in medicine and psychology, occupational therapy publications began to emerge that were specific to pediatrics. The first published assessment scale in pediatric occupational therapy appears to have been a daily living skill checklist for children with cerebral palsy that was printed in the *American Journal of Occupational Therapy* in 1950 (Reed & Sanderson, 1999). In the second edition of Willard & Spackman's *Principles of Occupational Therapy*, "children's play" was listed by McNary (1954, p. 16) as one of the activities that may be used by occupational therapists. At that time, pediatric practice in a hospital setting was described as helping the child adjust to the hospital, determining and aiding the

---

[1] For the original article in the newspaper that describes the opening of this playground in Chicago, see *http://tigger.uic.edu/htbin/cgiwrap/bin/urbanexp/main.cgi?file=viewer.ptt&mime=blank&doc=631&type=pdf*; for a slide show that includes slides of the playground's development, see *http://tigger.uic.edu/htbin/cgiwrap/bin/urbanexp/main.cgi?file=img/show_gallery.ptt&gallery=2*

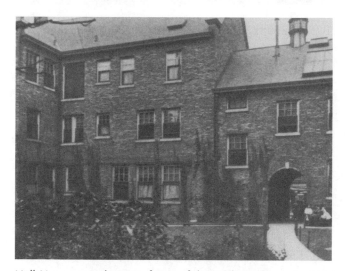

Hull House was the site of one of the earliest playgrounds in America.

HHYB-1907-0053-5539, Hull-House Yearbook (1907), University of Illinois at Chicago Library, Special Collections.

developmental sequence, and improving kinetic function. McNary discussed that play could be used to teach elements of self-care and to help the child adjust to being in the hospital. Toys were specifically mentioned as important treatment tools.

Gleave (1954) provided an early look at client-centered pediatric occupational therapy practice. She discussed the use of activities such as crafts, recreation (play), and music with children and specifically stressed the importance of the child's participation in choice making throughout her chapter, stating "the child should have an opportunity to contribute to the program" (p. 164), and "the development of play interests in the child must be considered" (p. 164). In addition, Gleave (1954) mentioned the usefulness of crafts specifically because they allowed the child "unlimited opportunities for self expression and permit[ed] the child to pursue his natural interests" (p. 164). Therefore, some of the ideas of client-centered pediatric practice are not new but are part of the occupational therapy tradition.

Although some of the concepts of client-centered therapy existed in early pediatric practice, the views on play were somewhat different from what they are now. Early in the history of occupational therapy, play was generally used merely as a diversion for the sick or ill child. Later it was primarily used as a method to develop other skills. The idea that play itself is important and and worthy of our time in intervention without an alternative agenda is a more modern perspective.

The emergence of play as an important activity in occupational therapy worthy of study can be traced back

to A. Jean Ayres (1963, 1964, 1971, 1972) and Mary Reilly (1974). Although the work of Ayres in the development of sensory integration theory was not specific only to play, she highlighted the importance of play in the way intervention is delivered. Child-directed play is key to Ayres' Sensory Integration approach[2], and Ayres' respect for children and the value she placed on play is clear in all of her work. She believed, similar to others of the time, that play reflected learning (and sensory integration), that children had an inner drive to play, and that play could be used to enhance learning (and sensory integration). These beliefs were similar to those held by Mary Reilly and were common during this time period. As you may recall from Chapter One, during this time period, these authors would have been exposed to the works of Piaget (1962) and others who considered play as reflective of and important for development. In addition, the importance of motivation for activity had been written about by White (1959), and these ideas also influenced Ayres and Reilly (Schaaf, Merrill, & Kinsella, 1987).

The first published text in occupational therapy specifically about play was edited by Reilly in 1974. This instrumental work of Mary Reilly and her students (Florey, 1971; Knox, 1974; Takata, 1974) provided our profession with a base of knowledge specific to our field. Reilly proposed three hierarchical stages of play development— exploratory, competency, and achievement—and suggested that play allowed learning and mastery to occur for the child. Florey described play as a learning process and identified the importance of play in natural environments. Florey also spoke about the importance of the environment to either inhibiting or facilitating play, and the impact of disability on play. Takata similarly believed play and development were inextricably linked and that play therefore followed a predictable sequence of development. She created a taxonomy of play based on age and developmental level (**Figure 2-2**) that is still used today. These early researchers created initial assessments of play that used both observation (Knox, 1974) and interview (Takata, 1974). Knox's Preschool Play Scale was used to study play in different populations in a small group of studies on play that were carried out over the next 15–20 years. For example, play behaviors were compared between children who were and were not hospitalized (Kielhofner, Barris, Bauer, Shoestock, & Walker, 1983), between children who had and had not been abused (Howard, 1986), between children of differing socioeconomic status (von Zuben, Crist &

---

[2] see *http://www.siglobalnetwork.org/*

Figure 2-2   Takata's (1974) Taxonomy of Play

- *Birth to 2 years:* sensorimotor
- *Two to 4 years:* symbolic and simple constructive
- *Four to 7 years:* dramatic, complex constructive, and pre-game
- *Seven to 12 years:* games
- *Twelve to 16 years:* recreational

Adapted from Takata, 1974

Mayberry, 1991), and between children with and without autism (Restall & Magill-Evans, 1994).

During the time after Reilly's book, however, play appeared to hold little interest for occupational therapy researchers because few published studies on play were completed. As a group, these few studies reported above generally examined one aspect of play—the type, form, or category—or they examined characteristics of play to measure developmental skills in other areas. Play was not considered for the sake of play but because it could influence development in other areas. Over time, new concepts of play began to be considered, and authors began writing about play in a new way, influenced by new models of occupational therapy practice and, in turn, influencing practice.

■ NEW CONCEPTS OF PLAY IN OCCUPATIONAL THERAPY

In 1993, Bundy stated, "it is telling that we who claim that play and leisure are a primary lifelong human occupation and who make it our business to assess occupation, have contributed so little to the existing theoretical and practical knowledge base of play" (p. 219). She promoted the idea that play and leisure should be an explicit goal of occupational therapy intervention and prompted the profession to examine play as an occupation rather than just a means to another end. Echoing Kielhofner and Barris (1984), Bundy began to critique the then available assessments of play. She believed it was much more important to measure whether or not a child could do what he or she wanted to do than to try to determine a developmental play age.

Throughout the 1990s, Bundy developed both a model of playfulness and assessment tools to measure aspects of her model. She suggested that playfulness is a style of approaching activities that transcends the activity itself. Playfulness is an attitude manifested in joy, flexibility, and spontaneity. Her current Model of Playfulness (Skard &

Bundy, 2008) proposes three primary elements that must be present for playfulness to exist: intrinsic motivation, internal control, and freedom to suspend reality. Intrinsic motivation means that the focus of the activity is on the process, not the product, and that the player chooses the activity because he or she wants to do it. Internal control is a characteristic of playfulness that allows the player to decide whom to play with, what to play with, and how and when to play. A child who is playful also has the freedom to suspend reality, the ability to pretend and take risks. This model and the research that surrounded its development prompted a resurgence of interest in play in occupational therapy.

This renewed interest in play resulted in the publication of the first comprehensive texts on play in occupational therapy since Reilly's work (Chandler, 1997; Parham & Fazio, 1996). Researchers in occupational science must also be given credit for the revival of interest in play in occupational therapy. More recent writings in occupational therapy remind us that play is an integral part of the human experience (Parham, 1996, 2007), not merely a vehicle for enhancing other skills. This new literature suggests that play may be important for the quality of life of the child and for enhancing health. Occupational therapists have been refocused on play as an occupation rather than as a skill. If occupational therapists seek to understand play as an occupation, they must examine the meaning it provides in people's lives and study play as it occurs in real contexts.

Play as an Occupation

The Missing Piece of Meaning

Clark and colleagues (1991) suggested that occupations have *form, function*, and *meaning*. In terms of play, the form includes specific play activities that are commonly accepted and named. Many authors categorize the forms of play as discussed in Chapter One. A consideration of the form of play also includes the examination of the particular characteristics of play.

As discussed in Chapter One (see "Why Do Children Play?"), the *function* of play is still hotly debated. Although there is not yet a strong research base to support this assertion, our belief in occupational therapy is that play has significance for the mental health and quality of life of the individual who plays. The function of play for humans and other nonhuman species may be to promote flexibility, creativity, problem solving, and adaptation to novel situations in the environment, but as occupational therapists, we also believe in the power of play to make life joyful for a child and to enhance well-being for both children and adults.

The *meaning* of play for a child is something occupational therapists are just beginning to investigate (Miller & Kuhaneck, 2008; Pollack et al., 1997; Spitzer, 2003a, 2003b, 2004), but there is no doubt that childhood play is meaningful. Ask any adult about their favored childhood playthings or favorite play activities, and lengthy emotion-laden descriptions can ensue. There are many potential meanings of play for an individual, and likely these meanings will change over time with development. Some may find play meaningful, particularly for the challenge it provides and the mastery that it entails. Others may find play meaningful for the social experiences it engenders. Others may find play meaningful for the competition. Still others may find meaning in the sensory experience or in the imaginative fantasy that can occur in play. The meaning attributed to play may be as varied and unique as the individual players.

Learning Activity

Ask 5–10 adults of varying ages and backgrounds (cultural, socioeconomic, etc.) about their favorite playthings or their most vivid remembrances of pretending as a child. Listen for the emotion in the storytelling and the significance the memory might hold for the individual. Ask the individual to articulate why that play was important to him or her. Then ask a variety of children from ages 4 to 18 the same questions and compare the responses. Does this influence your perception of the importance of play for your practice with clients?

Research on the meaning of play for children can include asking them about their perceptions directly, but this may preclude the gathering of information from our clients with disabilities who lack the language to communicate with us in this way. A different approach is required to become informed regarding the meaning of play for children without language. Spitzer (2003a, 2003b, 2004) used the qualitative method of participant observation in her research to understand the occupations of children with autism. A sample of five children aged 3 and 4 years participated in the study. None of the children had sufficient language to adequately explain why they were engaging in their chosen activities. Most occupational therapists can call to mind a child with autism who engages in an activity we would not readily name as play but is one that seems very gratifying and enjoyable to that child. Over a course of months, Spitzer was able to begin to infer the meaning of the seemingly unusual occupations of these children with autism. Spitzer's work suggests that careful observation of the "what" and the "how" of an activity may allow us to attempt to understand the "why." She was able to infer very different meanings of the child's activities for the child from those an adult might have initially described on brief examination. She suggested that to infer the meaning of the activities of children when language is not an available method of sharing meaning, adults must "bridge the gaps." Specifically, she recommended that adults suspend adult judgments, assume that the child's actions are meant as communication, share in activities with the child to try to understand their meaning, follow what the child is doing, and engage in the activity themselves to examine the sensations the activity provides.

Recent work has attempted to examine the meaning of play for children by asking them directly. Children have rarely been asked why they choose what they play. If one asks children, their answers are quite enlightening. To our knowledge, four studies have been completed specifically asking children about their definitions of play, their play preferences, and their rationale for their choices (Caiazzo, Sarra, Vechionne, Miller, & Miller Kuhaneck, 2008; Miller & Kuhaneck, 2008; Pollack et al., 1997; Skar, 2002), and another asked children with disabilities about their participation in activities including play (Heah, Case, McGuire, & Law, 2007).

Children who were interviewed about their choices in play and their definitions of play suggested a variety of elements that made an activity play for them (Miller & Kuhaneck, 2008). When asked why they prefer certain play activities, children generally responded with the word "fun." Several categories emerged for the children in terms of what made something fun: activity characteristics, relational characteristics, child characteristics, and contextual characteristics. The children spoke of their pleasurable emotions during play, their idea that play was the opposite of boredom (suggesting the importance of novelty for play), the importance of social engagement for play, and the need for play activities to have the appropriate level of challenge. Although the children reported highly individualized choices of what they considered favored play, the common thread was that their preferred choices were all considered fun.

As a follow-up to the qualitative study of Miller and Kuhaneck (2008), a survey of 528 children aged 8–11 was completed (Caiazzo et al., 2008). Survey questions were developed based on the model created in the qualitative work. The survey results supported the model with a larger variety of children. Children indicated a strong preference for active play, outdoor play, play with peers, and a medium challenge level in their play. In answering one open-ended question regarding why they liked to play their favorite activity, 35% used the word "fun," 21% mentioned the high level of physical activity, 21% mentioned either the challenge of the activity as attractive or the ability to successfully meet the challenge provided by the activity, and 18% mentioned companionship.

Research is also beginning to examine the meaning of play for children with disabilities. In one study, 20 adolescents with and without disabilities were asked about the meaning of play (Pollack et al., 1997). Similar to the typically developing children who focused on fun as the reason for their play, these teens also spoke about play using the word "fun" and described the characteristics of the activity as play rather than the specific activity itself. The most important factor in their concept of fun was the participation in the activity with peers. They discussed that an activity could be both work and play based on the location, the time, and the purpose. The aspect of choice was very important in determining whether something was work or play, as was the amount of spontaneity. The children with disabilities mentioned their physical limitations but did not dwell on them. However, psychosocial barriers were mentioned, such as the difficulty making friends with whom to play.

Heah et al. (2007) asked children with disabilities about their experiences with participation in the community. These children also mentioned the importance of fun in their decisions for what activities to participate in and whether to continue their participation. They also wanted to feel successful in their endeavors, which to the children often meant "beating" someone at something or just being able to do something well. The children in this study also believed being with others was very important.

Play in Natural Environments

Whereas much of the play research in other fields documented children's play in laboratory settings, occupational scientists proposed that play be examined as it occurs in its natural environments. Occupational therapy researchers therefore examined children's play in typical contexts. Primeau (1998) examined play as it occurred within the home during the typical day-to-day routines of 10 families with preschool-age children. She was interested in the way in which parents orchestrated their child's play while completing their own household occupations. Through extensive participant observation and interviewing, she found that parents used two strategies to play with their child: segregation and inclusion. Segregation strategies were used when the parent removed him- or herself from the child's play or removed the child from his or her housework. Inclusion occurred when the parent created some way of playing with the child while in the midst of completing household chores or work. Primeau suggested that these two different strategies lead to either play interspersed with work or play embedded in work. She found that play was more likely to be embedded in child-care tasks than in other household tasks and that this play during child care often facilitated the task's completion. In addition, she found that during household tasks, when inclusive strategies were used, scaffolded play often occurred. This scaffolded play allowed parents to involve their children in the household task and assist their child in completing the task as independently as possible. Parents modified activities, provided verbal or physical guidance, or completed the most difficult steps while allowing the child to complete the portions he or she could do independently. Primeau's findings are important in considering play versus work. She found that for many of the families, work and play were often blended.

Knox (1997) also examined children's play in the natural environment of the classroom. A child brings a particular way of playing, or "play style," to any play episode. In her dissertation, Knox (1997) examined the play styles of children and considered questions of the uniqueness of play style, the influence of environmental factors on play style, and the ability to differentiate play from nonplay based on play style. Six children were observed, and different patterns of play style were demonstrated among the six children. The children were observed in different settings and over time, and influences of setting on play style were reported to be substantial. Knox (1997) also described preschool children's play style as the attitudes, approaches, and preferences brought to a play activity. Her research suggests that the children's approach to both play and nonplay tasks may have been similar. Knox's (1997) interactive model of play, which developed from this study, considers both the child and the environment and has implications for occupational therapy intervention. The model guides the therapist to consider not only what the child brings to the play experience but also what the environment affords. This research also suggests the importance of considering a child's play preference in designing interventions based on play.

Another study of play in natural environments was conducted internationally and reminded U.S. occupational therapists that our belief that play is a child's *primary* occupation may not be a universally held belief (Bazyk, Stalnaker, Llerena, Ekelman, & Bazyk, 2003). In a qualitative examination of the play of 20 Mayan children in five families, the researchers found that play was allowed if it did not interfere with adult work but was not encouraged by adults as play, as it often is here in the United States. However, the authors' findings did support play as a universal desire of children because these children somehow found ways to play within their daily activities.

Contextual Influences

As newer occupational therapy models have stressed the importance of examining the contexts in which occupations occur, occupational therapists have begun to examine the contextual features that influence play as well. Although early studies of play in occupational therapy hinted that the environment could impact play and playfulness (Kielhofner et al., 1983), later work has more systematically examined the influences of environment. Knox (1997) specifically examined the environmental features that influenced play style, and Skard and Bundy (2008) created an assessment tool that examines the environmental supports for playfulness. Certain environments lend themselves toward certain play, and a good fit between the player and the play environment is important for playfulness to emerge (Skard & Bundy, 2008). Important environmental features that support play and playfulness include physical safety, space for play, time for play, availability of developmentally appropriate and preferred play materials, and appropriate social interaction with either peers or adults.

One extremely important contextual feature may be the parent's beliefs and attitudes toward play and his or her style of playing. It is likely that having a playful, engaging parent encourages playful behaviors in a child. There is a small body of research examining parental attitudes toward child's play and the relationship between these attitudes and actual child behaviors and playfulness (Porter & Bundy, 2001) (see also Chapters Four and Nine). Studies have suggested that supportive maternal play behavior may encourage object play (Roach, Barratt, Miller, & Leavitt, 1998), and there is some evidence that play is more developmentally competent when an adult caregiver is present (Daunhauer, Coster, Tickle-Degnen, & Cermak,

2007). Some authors therefore promote playful parenting (Cohen, 2001), and some intervention programs promote play and playfulness for child development (Parent-Child Home Program).[3]

Research exists on the benefits of intensive play-based programming, particularly with children with autism and developmental disabilities, and there is research suggesting that children with autism respond better to sillier and more playful adults (Gillett & LeBlanc, 2007; Kasari, Freeman, & Paparella, 2006; Lifter, 2000; Nadel, Martini, Field, Escalona, & Lundy, 2008; Solomon, Necheles, Ferch, & Bruckman, 2007; Stahmer, 1995; Thorp, Stahmer, & Schreibman, 1995; Wolfberg & Schuler, 1993). However, little research exists documenting the ability to specifically increase *playfulness* in parents or the effects of increasing playfulness in parents. There is not yet a fully developed assessment tool to measure parent playfulness specifically. There is research to support that parent *responsiveness* is important for child playfulness (Chiarello, Huntington, & Bundy, 2006), but responsiveness is not identical to playfulness. Thus, it may be important to consider the playfulness of the adults in a child's life, but much more research in this area is needed.

■ CONCLUSION

The profession's views on play have changed since its inception, and there has been a resurgence of interest in occupational therapy research in the realm of play. New conceptions of both occupations in general and play specifically have challenged us as occupational therapists to

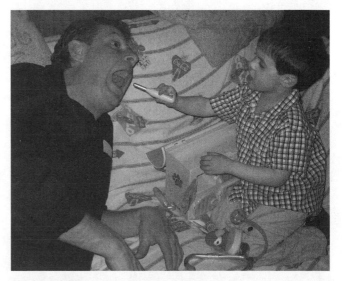

Playful adults may support and encourage more competent play in children.

[3] see *http://www.parent-child.org/aboutus/index.html*

alter our views on the function of play and to begin to examine the meaning of play for children. Occupational therapy's emphasis on client-centered care pushes us to consider the play preferences of the children we serve and to incorporate play and playfulness into our evaluations and interventions on a more consistent basis. Although we still have much to learn, occupational therapists are closer than ever to understanding the importance of play for our clients. As we learned in Chapter One, there is a growing acceptance of the importance of play and playfulness for children and adults in diverse professions outside of occupational therapy (Ginsburg et al., 2007). This suggests that now, more than ever, we must assert ourselves as a profession able and willing to help children to play.

In this day and age of accountability and focus on reimbursement, in certain situations, some therapists may believe play is not important enough to warrant our time. Therapists may be pushed to focus on handwriting, dressing or feeding skills, or other more "worklike" areas of function. However, the premise of this entire book is that for the occupational therapist working with a child with a disability, play should be evaluated and included as a *primary* goal of intervention and that work and play should not be segmented. We must express to those on our team and those who employ us that play *is* important and is worthy of our time (Ginsburg et al., 2007). These first two chapters provide the information to make well-founded arguments in support of play in general and in therapy for our clients.

Section Two
The Skills and Tools You Need...

Examining Play in Our Pediatric Clients: Formal Assessments and Activity Analysis

After completing this chapter the reader will

1. Recognize the variety of formal assessment tools available for play assessment in occupational therapy.

2. Articulate the importance of naturalistic and clinical observation in examining play.

3. Recognize the importance of activity analysis as a form of ongoing assessment in pediatric occupational therapy.

4. Relate the history of activity analysis to our current emphasis on its use.

5. Explain the similarities and differences between types of activity analysis.

6. Describe the process of completing a general and client-focused activity analysis.

7. Demonstrate the ability to complete a general activity analysis using the form provided.

8. Describe the types of goals occupational therapists may write in regard to play.

> *You can discover more about a person in an hour of play than in a year of conversation.*
> —Plato

The examination of play is a critical piece of any pediatric occupational therapy evaluation. As discussed in Chapters One and Two, to assess play as an occupation, there are many aspects to be considered in addition to merely what and how the child plays. The differing features of play that must be included in our evaluation suggest the use of multiple methods of assessment. There are many from which to choose. There are a variety of formal and structured play assessment tools. There are parent questionnaires and parent and child interviews. And, more important, a therapist may observe a child playing in person or via videotape, in a natural context, with typical materials, and with typical playmates. However, applying activity analysis during naturalistic observations may be our most successful method of assessing play. This chapter discusses each form of assessment, providing an overview of the strategies available to us and focusing on the use of activity analysis in pediatric practice. In addition, to highlight the importance placed on activity analysis in occupational therapy with pediatric clients, we document the long history of this tool in practice. Finally, we consider goal writing for play as one outcome of a thorough play evaluation in children in need of occupational therapy services.

■ EVALUATION OF PLAY

Although many occupational therapists profess that they believe play is important, it appears that few actually formally evaluate it (Couch, Deitz, & Kanny, 1998). This, in part, may be due to the types of play assessments currently available, or it may be that in the act of assessing play, therapists believe they are altering it, changing it from its most natural form. It may also be due to external considerations such as insurance reimbursement, constraints placed by school administrators, or a variety of other reasons we *believe* do not allow us to focus on play. Whatever the reason, for those reading this text, we hope you will begin to evaluate play more frequently and formally, just as you evaluate motor skills and other areas of performance in children.

In Chapter One, we discussed the "w" questions of play in a general fashion, but therapists can and should answer the "w" questions of play for each child. We need to know what the child plays, what the child likes to play or wants to play, and if that is different from what he or she is able to play. We need to know who the child's playmates are, and when and where they play. We need to know why the child plays what he or she plays. By observing the play of the child and asking yourself or the child about why he or she is playing this thing, you may find some important insights (Spitzer, 2003a, 2003b).

To answer the different "w" questions, we may use a variety of methods. Just as we often use multiple tools and methods to evaluate activities of daily living or motor skills, we may need many tools and methods to examine play. Information should be gathered about the child through typical evaluation methods, finding out about the child's skills and abilities and developmental level cognitively and physically in relation to his or her ability to play. During an evaluation of play, occupational therapists may use formal assessment tools, record review, parent questionnaires and interviews, observation in a variety of natural or clinical environments, and, as we highlight in this chapter, activity analysis. First, let us consider the range of formal assessment tools now available to us in pediatric occupational therapy.

Play Assessment Tools

Many therapists, particularly those newer to pediatric practice, can benefit from having a formal assessment tool as a guide. Although it is beyond the scope of this text to thoroughly describe each assessment, we believe these tools can play a useful and important role in examining play. Most of these tools examine only certain aspects of play, and therefore, most are not thorough enough on their own. **Table 3-1** lists the currently available play assessments that examine how children play. This text is not meant to provide a comprehensive discussion of the use of formal assessments of play. Readers are referred to other texts such as Parham and Fazio (2007) for a more in-depth consideration of formal assessments of play.

In addition to those tools listed, another important component of the occupational therapy evaluation is to determine the child's preferences for play and the meaningfulness of the activities for the child (the what and the why of their play). Interviews and questionnaires can be very helpful in this process but must be tailored to the child's developmental level. Several tools have been developed to assist in this process: Children's Assessment of Participation and Enjoyment (King et al., 2004), Preferences for Activities of Children (King et al., 2004), Perceived Efficacy and Goal Setting System (Missiuna, Pollock, & Law, 2004), Kid Play Profile (Henry, 2000, 2008), and Preteen Play Profile (Henry, 2008). The Play Activity Questionnaire (Finegan, Niccols, Zacher, & Hood, 1991) examines play preferences as well and has been used in some studies of gendered play.

Informal Play Assessment

In the case of young children or children with limited communication, alternative approaches must be used. Family and caregiver interviews and questionnaires potentially can help in identifying the child's interests (Bryze, 2008; Burke, Schaaf, & Hall, 2008; Takata, 1974); however, caregiver report alone may not accurately indicate a child's preference (Reid, DiCarlo, Schepis, Hawkins, & Stricklin, 2003). Observations and reading of the child's cues can provide indicators of the child's interests and desires (Holloway, 2008; Knox, 2008; Spitzer, 2003a, 2003b). The communication strategies described in Chapter Four, as well as assistive technology devices, can be used to help a child express his or her preferences (Lane & Mistrett, 2008).

In the gathering of information to answer the "w" questions of play for each child, you may choose not to use any formal assessment tools at all. You may decide to observe the child playing and interview the child and parent in an attempt to answer your questions. In cases such as this, it may be helpful to have a list of questions as a reminder. **Figure 3-1** provides some questions to ask in regard to the child's play preferences and the meaning of play for the child. There are questions that provide information in all areas (who, what, where, when, and why).

While asking these questions and gathering information, it may be helpful for you to use a grid, such as the one in **Figure 3-2**, to organize the information being gathered. A copy of Figure 3-2 is available online at *http://www.jbpub.com* so that you may use the form as many times as you need it. Answers to the questions in Figure 3-1 can be listed in the appropriate areas with symbols or notations indicating whether there is a problem in that area. For example, you could use **+** to designate a strength, **−** to designate needs, and ✓ to indicate which areas may require further evaluation or intervention.

Table 3-1   Available Assessments of Play Skills and Playfulness*

Play Assessment Tool	Authors	Tool Type	Description
Play History	Takata (1974); Taylor, Menarchek-Fetkovich, & Day (2000); Bryze (2008)	Semi-structured interview format with play observation	Examines a child's history of play, skills used during play, and choices made for play.
Preschool Play Scale	Knox (1974, 2008)	Play observation	Examines developmental skills demonstrated during play.
Play Assessment Scale	Fewell (1986)	Play observation	Examines child's play that demonstrates perceptual or conceptual skills or processes.
Playground Skills Test	Butcher (1991)	Play observation	Examines the motor skills and proficiency of children in elementary schools while out on the playground.
Trans-disciplinary Play Based Assessment	Linder (1993, 2000)	Play observation	Assesses four domains of child development: sensorimotor, emotional and social, communication and language, and cognition.
Test of Playfulness	Bundy (1997); Skard & Bundy (2008)	Play observation	Measures aspects of playfulness (intrinsic motivation, locus of control, and ability to suspend reality).
Assessment of Ludic Behavior	Ferland (1997)	Criterion referenced assessment of play behavior	Examines the child's play behaviors, play attitudes, and features of the environment that help or hinder play; for children with disabilities.
Pediatric Volitional Questionnaire	Geist & Kielhofner (1998)	Observation tool	Examines child's motivations during play in natural environments.
Test of Environmental Supportiveness	Bundy (1999); Hamm (2006); Skard & Bundy (2008)	Play observation	Rates elements of the environment that help or hinder playfulness.
Penn Interactive Peer Play Scale (PIPPS)	Hampton (1999)	Rating scale with versions for parents and teachers	Examines peer play.
Developmental Play Assessment	Lifter (2000)	Curriculum-based observation	Assesses children's play to enable the design of play intervention programs; designed for preschool-age children but can be adapted for older or younger children.
Play Observation Kit (POKIT)	Mogford-Bevan (2000)	Play observation with standard toys	Examines spontaneous interactive play.
Symbolic Play Test	Power & Radcliffe (2000)	Play observation with standard toys	Examines the cognitive skills of children aged 1–3 through play.
Parent Child Interaction Play Assessment Method	Smith (2000)	Observation measure	Examines unstructured play and response to parental commands.
Play Observation Scale	Rubin (2001)	Play observation	Measures the components of play outlined by Piaget, nested within the social categories of play as described by Parten.
Children's Playfulness Scale	Trevlas, Grammatikopoulos, Tsigilis, & Zachopoulou (2003)	Likert rating scale	Measures spontaneity, joy, and sense of humor.
Child-initiated Pretend Play Assessment (ChiPPA)	Stagnitti (2007)	Norm-referenced standardized assessment	Examines a child's imaginative or pretend play skills for children aged 3–7; measures how elaborate a child's play is and the child's ability to use symbols and self-initiate.

*Assessments are in order of the publication year of the first citation listed, and then within the same year are alphabetical by first author.

Data from sources listed in the table

Figure 3-1   Questions to Consider When Assessing a Child's Play Preferences

Goal: Determine what is fun for the child and why

Patterns, Persistence, and Preference
- What type of play does this child gravitate to if given free choice?
- What does the child say is his or her favorite play?
- What does this child do over and over again? Why might that be?

Child Characteristics
- What is the child's gender? Does this child seek out gendered activity choices?
- What is the child's age? Does this child seek out activities typical of this chronological age? Developmental age?

Activity Characteristics
- Is the preferred activity active or passive?
- What is the level of challenge the activity provides?
- Is it an attainable activity but not too easy?
- What are the sensory characteristics of the activity?

Match
- Is there a good match between the activity characteristics (level of challenge) and the child characteristics (level of skill and ability)?

Relational Characteristics
- With whom does the child like to play? Does this child play alone, with peers, with sibling(s), or with pets?
- Who decides what to play? Are choices shared?
- If playing with adults, are the adults playful?

Contextual Characteristics
- Where does this child prefer to play? Indoors or outdoors?
- Is there one location where play is more easily encouraged?
- What is available to play with?
- When does this child have time to play?

Emotions
- What makes this child laugh? What elicits emotion from this child?
- When is this child happiest?

Mastery
- Is there an improvement during play in emotion, choice making, intention, or interaction?
- Does the child indicate feelings of success or verbalize success?
- Is there an improvement in the child's skills and abilities during or after play?

Based on Miller & Miller-Kuhaneck (2008)

Figure 3-2   Grid Used to View the Answers to the Questions Posed in Figure 3-1

Patterns/Persistence/Preference	Child Characteristics	Activity Characteristics	Activity–Child Match
Stated preference:	Gender:	Active:	Challenge vs. child abilities:
		Challenge:	
Frequency:	Developmental:	Sensory:	

Relational Characteristics	Contextual Characteristics	Emotions	Mastery
Child playmates:	Where (indoors/ outdoors):	Laughs at:	Improvements during, through, or after play:
Adult playmates:	Availability of materials, space:	Most happy:	Experience of success:

Based on Miller & Miller-Kuhaneck (2008)

Assessment of Peer Relationships and Friendships

One aspect of a thorough evaluation of play is to examine the relationships between the who, what, where, when, and why of play. We must consider how a child's play affects with whom the child plays and how that may influence other aspects of his or her occupational performance. An important outcome for occupational therapy may be assisting a child in being able to play in order to form friendships with desired peers.

Research suggests the importance of shared play among children in creating peer culture and friendships (Elgas, Klein, Kantor, & Fernie, 1988; Goldman & Buysse, 2007; Whaley & Rubenstein, 1994). The ability of very young children to carefully imitate their peers in play is important in their early development of friendships (Whaley & Rubenstein, 1994). In many children with disabilities, physical limitations inhibit the ability to carefully imitate favored peers; in children with sensory integration dysfunction, deficits in motor planning may limit that ability as well. Occupational therapists should be attuned to the child's ability to specifically imitate others in play as more than merely a "play stage" (parallel play, associative play) to go through. Although in young children, imitation is frequently seen with many other individuals, in toddlers, "friend" imitation is often exact and leads to synchrony between friends (Whaley & Rubenstein, 1994). Other important features of early friendships include sharing, helping, separating from others in the friendship pair, and loyalty. Therapists can readily observe these characteristics of young friendships through play in natural settings.

Occupational therapists should be aware of the features of friendship that occur through play. We must evaluate our clients' ability to engage in peer play that fosters the growth of friendships and allows them access into the peer culture in which they are in. The importance of friendships for a child's well-being cannot be overstated (Antle, 2004; Goldman & Buysee, 2007; Hartup, 1996; Matheson, Olsen, & Weisner, 2007; Mulderji, 1997).

■ ACTIVITY ANALYSIS: A KEY METHOD OF ASSESSMENT

Although much information regarding play can be gathered via the use of formal play assessment tools and interviews with the parents and the child, it is also extremely important to observe the child completing actual play activities. One important method of play assessment is completed using the typical process of activity analysis,

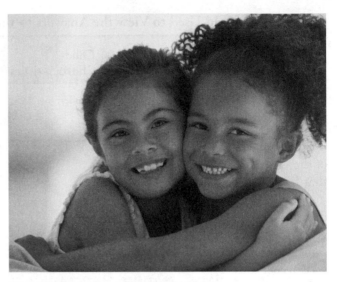

Friendships are important for well being.

which is the focus of the next section. We provide information regarding the historical development and evolution of activity analysis as an occupational therapy tool and suggest methods for completing general activity analysis and client-focused activity analysis that is focused on pediatric clients.

One of the earliest tools of the profession, and one of the most fundamental skills occupational therapists possess, is the ability to analyze activities. There have been multiple definitions of activity analysis throughout the history of occupational therapy. The common element within the definitions is the careful observation of an activity to identify the features of the activity that may be adapted and/or used therapeutically. Fidler and Velde (1999, p. 48) described activity analysis as follows:

> [A] process that assesses the elements or characteristics of an activity for the purpose of identifying and defining the dimensions of its performance requirements and its social and cultural significance and meanings. It is a process of looking at parts as these relate to the whole.

Mosey (1981, 1986) described activity analysis as the process of distinguishing the parts of an activity via careful observation to then select the most appropriate activities for use in intervention. Llorens (1993) added the dimension of client desires and motivations in her description of activity analysis. Our definition of activity analysis for this text is as follows: *a process of examining the essential elements of a task or activity to identify both its fundamental requirements and its opportunities for therapeutic use.*

Although the literature has incorporated first the Uniform Terminology (Cottrell, 1996) and, more recently, the Occupational Therapy Practice Framework (OTPF) in writings about activity analysis (American Occupational Therapy Association [AOTA], 2008; Crepeau, 2003; Hersch, Lamport, & Coffey, 2005), Fidler and Velde (1999) warned about the use of such documents to guide activity analysis. They stated that it was difficult to translate certain portions of the Uniform Terminology into the analysis of an activity. The same could be said of the OTPF. There are areas of the OTPF, for example, that focus on the client rather than the activity. More important, Fidler and Velde (1999) suggested that using documents such as the Uniform Terminology could lead therapists to miss the essential meaning of an activity or some essential aspect of the activity's character. In this text, we consider the OTPF where it is applicable, but the process we suggest for the general analysis of activities does not strictly follow its format or structures.

Some authors suggested that the process of activity analysis be renamed "occupation analysis" (Punwar, 2000), thus refocusing therapists on the aspect of consideration of the meaning of the activity for the client. We use the term "activity analysis" in this book. There are times when therapists use this process without connection to an individual making meaning of the task. One can do an activity analysis of bike riding, irrespective of who might be riding the bike or how meaningful the task could be to someone. Occupational therapists use activity analysis as a tool to understand the components of activities that can be used in therapeutic ways for their clients or that can be altered to allow their clients successful performance in desired activities.

Whatever one's definition of activity analysis, the purpose is the same. Activity analysis is used to "help one arrive at some understanding of the basic and fundamental...characteristics of a given activity" (Fidler & Fidler, 1963, p. 75) and to "arrive at an understanding of the activity's inherent qualities and characteristics, its meaning in and of itself, irrespective of a performer" (Fidler & Velde, 1999, p. 47). This knowledge then is used in the clinical reasoning process of the therapist to modify the activity or engage the client in the appropriate activity with the just-right challenge that provides therapeutic value and a match to the client's current capabilities. Part of this process is the ability to compare activity A with activity B to consider the features of each and determine which is best for a client to meet a particular goal.

Prior literature on activity analysis has divided it into different types (Crepeau, 2003; Hersch et al., 2005), and this text does so as well. Activity analysis is discussed in terms of general activity analysis and client-focused activity analysis. General activity analysis is the process through which occupational therapists learn to analyze specific activities in great detail. This type of activity analysis is often done by novice occupational therapists or therapists encountering a novel activity. Typically, a student will engage in an activity and then complete a full analysis for the express purpose of learning the process of activity analysis, whereas a therapist more skilled in the process will complete a general activity analysis to learn the essential features of a novel activity. General activity analysis allows us to determine the demands of an activity.

Client-focused activity analysis is a fundamental component of occupational therapy evaluation and intervention. During an evaluation, client-focused activity analysis allows a therapist to observe a client during the completion of a task and create hypotheses regarding the causes for a client's difficulties in performance, as well as hypotheses regarding how to alter or modify activities to increase client success and personal meaning. During client-focused activity analysis, the therapist must consider the activity in the context in which it is typically performed (Buckley & Poole, 2004).

The outcome of client-focused activity analysis, when combined with the knowledge generated through multiple trials of general activity analysis, is the therapist's ability to select an appropriate and meaningful therapeutic activity for a client; to adapt, alter, or modify an activity to allow a client to participate; and to rapidly grade components of activities to increase or decrease their difficulty for a client. For the purposes of this text, we use the terms "activity selection," "activity grading," and "activity modification" for the processes that follow activity analysis. We want to stress here that although practicing therapists typically do not complete formal general activity analyses and do not typically fill out lengthy paper forms, activity analysis is a crucial process in the ongoing intervention with any client. We constantly are reevaluating and completing informal activity analyses in our heads as needed to create the "just right challenge" for our clients. We consider this process to be essential to pediatric occupational therapy.

As a fundamental process in occupational therapy, we believe it is important to review the history of activity analysis. We include this history both to comment on how integral the process has become to occupational therapy and to honor the women and men who developed this valuable tool and contributed so importantly to our profession.

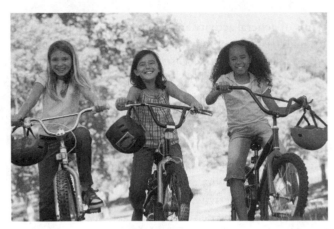

Occupational therapists can do a general activity analysis of bike riding, irrespective of who is riding, or a client-focused activity analysis to assess a client's specific strengths and difficulties in bike riding as a basis for treatment planning.

Brief History of Activity Analysis

The history of activity analysis in occupational therapy is a long one. From the beginning of the profession we have adapted knowledge from other fields to fit our needs, expanding the knowledge, and using it in new ways. In the case of activity analysis, the usage of knowledge was expanded in ways much greater than intended by the originators of the process. Two men associated with the concepts that led to the eventual emergence of activity analysis in occupational therapy are Frederick Taylor and Frank Gilbreth (Gilbreth 1904; Nadworny, 1957; Taylor, 1904). Both men were involved in the field of management, and both were ultimately interested in improving the efficiency of workers and the productivity of human labor (Nadworny, 1957). Taylor, the "Father of Scientific Management," is best known for the use of time study, recording the time needed to complete tasks with a stop-watch, with the ultimate goal of "increasing output per unit of human effort" (Taylor, 1904, p. 86). Gilbreth, a contemporary of Taylor's, was also interested in increasing worker productivity but believed that the way to achieve this end was to analyze work methods and motions to achieve economy of effort. He therefore focused on fatigue study and motion study using photographic film analysis to carefully observe the methods and motions workers used while performing their tasks (Barnes, 1949; Gilbreth, 1904; Nadworny, 1957). Gilbreth advocated surveying multiple people performing the same task to systematically examine differences and determine the one best way (i.e., most efficient way) of completing the activity. As early as 1904, Gilbreth was labeling this type of analysis a science, calling motion study "the science of determining and perpetuating the

scheme of perfection; the performing of the one best way to do work" (pp. 273–274).

Gilbreth and his wife were the first authors to publish information linking motion study specifically to work with the handicapped. In their papers, "The Re-Education of the Crippled Soldier" and "Motion Study for Crippled Soldiers," presented at conferences in 1915, 1916, and 1917 (Spriegel & Myers, 1953), the Gilbreths discussed how their studies of efficient methods could and should be transferred to the education of the wounded soldiers returning from war. These writings did not mention occupational therapy specifically, but their statements sounded quite similar to the philosophy of occupational therapy that was developing during the same time period. For example, the Gilbreths stated the importance of "arousing interest in the discovery, invention, or adaptation of devices that will make it possible for the [individual with a disability] not only to have a productive and paying occupation but also to 'fit back' into all of the ordinary activities of daily life" (Spriegel & Myers, 1953, p. 280). They also spoke about the way in which motion study created solutions and inventions necessary to allow soldiers to relearn and complete desired tasks. They discussed all aspects of activity analysis as occupational therapists currently use it: adapting methods to the soldier, choosing appropriate activities for the soldier based on what he could do, and modifying or adapting activities for the individual soldier. In these early writings, one can see the beginnings of activity analysis as occupational therapists still use it today.

The Gilbreths were quite influential in early occupational therapy. Mr. Gilbreth influenced the work of both Barton and Dunton, the first two presidents of the National Society for the Promotion of Occupational Therapy, and he presented his work at the new society's first annual meeting, where the influential founders of the profession were present (Creighton, 1992; Licht, 1967). A paper by Mrs. Gilbreth was presented in absentia at the initial meeting of the Society in 1917 at Consolation House (Licht, 1967). The ideas of the Gilbreth's thus spread throughout our early occupational therapy leaders.

Activity Analysis in Occupational Therapy

Not surprisingly, because activity analysis emerged from motion analysis in management, early discussions of this process in occupational therapy focused heavily on the analysis of *motions* for rehabilitation of clients. The first publication that discussed activity analysis with consideration of physical and social-emotional aspects of performance was disseminated in 1925 by Haas. Haas focused on therapists' careful consideration of which activity to choose for a patient because just "being busy is not necessarily therapeutic" (Haas, 1925, p. 25). In Haas's book, written for therapists working in the field of mental health, the term "activity analysis" is not used specifically, but the author described the therapeutic application of crafts and processes similar to our current conception of activity adaptation and grading specifically for clients whose difficulties were mental more than physical.

Although motion analysis continued to be important, the cognitive, sensory–perceptual, and psychological facets of activity became more routinely included in activity analysis as a variety of frames of reference were delineated in occupational therapy (Creighton, 1992; Fidler & Fidler, 1963; Llorens, 1973). Fidler, a strong advocate and passionate occupational therapist who often wrote about mental health issues, proposed an outline for activity analysis that carefully examined the psychodynamic aspects of the activity for the client (Fidler & Fidler, 1963). These aspects are listed in **Figure 3-3**.

As occupational therapy's knowledge base grew and our own theoretical orientations developed, activity analysis began to be linked with specific frames of reference. Llorens (1973, 1986) described different forms of activity analysis, highlighting the aspects of the activity that needed to be considered in relation to the particular frame of reference chosen. For example, when using Ayres' sensory integration frame of reference, the sensory qualities of the activity would be specifically examined. This aspect of activity analysis is discussed further in Chapters Five and Six. Recent history has adapted the formats and processes of activity analysis to new occupational therapy terminology and concepts. For example, Hersch and colleagues (2005) and Buckley and Poole (2004) promoted a process for activity analysis that has integrated the OTPF (AOTA, 2008). With the increased emphasis on consideration of context throughout occupational therapy, both works consider contextual features of activities as well.

Training of Students in Activity Analysis

Early records of occupational therapy from the military suggest that activity analysis was first used and taught to reconstruction aides during World War I. The early military training for these occupational therapy aides focused on a variety of specific crafts and motion analysis of each. The social-emotional or psychological impact of activities did not yet appear to be a strong consideration in training and intervention.[1] However, a large variety of crafts

were taught, suggesting that military educational practice considered it important to have a variety of activities available to allow for individual preferences and needs. An examination of the curriculum changes between the 6-month occupational therapy course at Walter Reed in 1924–1925 to the 9-month course taught in 1932–1933 shows the increased emphasis on the use of activities in treatment and the increased focus on activity analysis as well (McDaniel, n.d.).

Early curricula in occupational therapy outside of the military were highly varied, and no standards of education existed until 1924 (Colman, 1992). Even then, the standards adopted were minimum standards, which were very flexible and had little real enforcement. Much debate occurred in our early years regarding the content and the focus of occupational therapy education (Colman, 1990, 1992). The term "activity analysis" does not appear to be specifically mentioned in curriculum in our early years. The American Medical Association, in their "Essentials of an Acceptable School of Occupational Therapy" (1943), recommended first 25, and then 30, semester hours of instruction in a variety of therapeutic activities, but there was no specification of courses in activity analysis per se. In the 1950s, the military training of occupational therapists included in their discussions and demonstrations "the adaptations of activities for patient treatment and the analysis of activities for interest, exercise, and motion potential (fig. 137)."[2]

An increased emphasis on the medical model, with a concurrent decrease in emphasis on specific activities in training for occupational therapy, was evident in the 1965 essentials and the curriculum study completed in the early 1960s that recommended deemphasizing traditional arts and crafts (Kearney, 2004). In the 1970s, the first indication of the importance of training students to use activity analysis as a tool surfaced in the Essentials (AOTA, 1975; Kearney, 2004). According to the essentials developed in the 1970s, upon completion of an accredited occupational therapy program, a student should be able to complete activity analysis and relate the specific components of tasks to the needs of a client (AOTA, 1975; Kearney, 2004). Our current standard in occupational therapy (B.2.7) states that students must "Exhibit the ability to analyze tasks relative to areas of occupation, performance skills, performance patterns, activity demands, context(s), and client factors to formulate an intervention plan." (Accreditation Council for Occupational Therapy Education, 2008)

---

[1] see *http://history.amedd.army.mil/default_index2.html*

[2] see *http://history.amedd.army.mil/default_index2.html*

Figure 3-3   Fidler and Fidler's (1963) Outline for Activity Analysis Overview

1. *Motions:* Are the motions required passive, aggressive (hammering, banging), or destructive? Are the motions small or large? Do they require precision? Are they repetitive?

2. *Procedures:* What technical knowledge is required? Are there few or multiple steps? What new learning is required? What delays or postponements are required or possible?

3. *Materials and equipment:* What resistance is provided? Are materials pliable and flexible, or controllable?

4. *Creativity and originality:* How much creativity and expression is allowable in this activity? How do materials and supplies support or hinder creativity and expression?

5. *Symbols:* What may the materials and procedures symbolize or represent for an individual?

6. *Hostility and aggressiveness:* What characteristics of the activity provide an outlet for expression of hostility and aggression?

7. *Destructiveness:* What characteristics of the activity are destructive or may symbolize destruction?

8. *Control:* How in control of the activity is the performer? How much dependence on others is required? What limits are created by the activity or the materials and equipment?

9. *Predictability:* How predictable are the results of actions throughout the activity? How do the activities, materials, and methods reduce chances of failure? How can assistance and guidance be offered to increase predictability?

10. *Narcissism:* What opportunities are available for self-indulgence in this activity? Does the end product allow for monetary compensation or acknowledgment?

11. *Gender identification:* Is there a specific association with one gender for this activity?

12. *Dependency:* To what extent does this activity require or provide opportunities for being dependent on another?

13. *Infantilism:* What is the extent of actual or symbolic infantile activity, such as sucking, blowing, smearing, collecting, or possessing?

14. *Reality testing:* To what extent does this activity require or provide for clear standards or processes? Is reproduction of a sample required rather than free creativity?

15. *Self-identification:* To what extent can the performer identify his or her own efforts and contributions to the outcome or end product?

16. *Independence:* How does this activity provide for or require opportunities for independent planning and individual responsibility for success?

17. *Group relations:* How does this activity allow for or require cooperation and interdependence with others?

Data from Fidler & Fidler, 1963

Summary

Although the term "activity analysis" did not appear in our curriculum essentials until fairly recently, and the emphasis over time has shifted, clearly throughout our history, occupational therapists have been taught to use and examine meaningful activities in our interventions. Activity analysis, originally adapted from other fields, became a mainstay of our profession and one of our most important tools.

In working with clients, activity analysis becomes second nature to the seasoned occupational therapist. However, it is a skill that must be learned, and it takes practice to become adept. So, with this historical knowledge in hand, let us now turn to how to do an activity analysis.

Process of General Activity Analysis

Although a multitude of variables need to be considered during a general activity analysis, the steps to completing one are relatively simple[3] and can be used with any activity; however, thoroughness is necessary. The process for

[3] Many have written about the process of completing an activity analysis, and as stated by Buckley and Poole (2004), it is often difficult to determine where specific ideas originated. In creating our format and writing this chapter, many authors' works, were included, but much of the work comes from the writings of Gail Fidler and the information from Gayle Thompson's courses in activity analysis at Boston University in the late 1980s. The works of Buckley and Poole, Llorens, and Hersch, Lamport, and Coffey were also reviewed.

a general activity analysis is to engage in an activity until one has a good understanding of what the activity entails, describe the activity on paper, and list all of its steps. Next, one considers all aspects of the activity and the context within which the activity occurs. See **Figure 3-4** for a listing of the steps in the process of a general activity analysis, and **Appendix 3-1** for an activity analysis format with instructions. A blank activity analysis form is provided for you online at *http://www.jbpub.com.*

Client-Focused Activity Analysis

Once an occupational therapist has mastered the art of completing general activity analyses, the next task is to integrate that skill into practice with clients. Skill with activity analysis is useful for practitioners in their initial evaluations of client performance and throughout client intervention. The difference between the general and client-focused activity analysis is that when completing a client-focused activity analysis, the therapist must consider information not only about the activity and the specific context but also about the client. Often, this information is gathered during the initial evaluation as the therapist creates the occupational profile (AOTA, 2008). Using activity analysis while observing a specific client completing a specific activity in an evaluation or treatment allows the occupational therapist to determine what aspects of the activity are difficult for the client and why.

In a client-focused activity analysis, the chosen activity will reflect the roles, habits, routines, and preferences of the client. With young children or children with severe communication difficulties, however, sometimes the family may need to assist in this determination. Although it may be impossible to question the child about the meaning of

---

Learning Activities

View the video clips of children bike riding and observe children you know bike riding. Observe for similarities and differences. What essential elements of the activity are the same for every individual? Which elements change based on factors such as the context (hill vs. flat), the equipment (training wheels vs. none), or the age of the child or other child characteristics?

Examine the sample activity analysis provided (**Appendix 3-2**) and then complete a general activity analysis of an activity of your choice. Follow all steps of the process and complete the blank form provided for you. The form is available for you online at *www.jbpub.com.*

---

the activity, the enjoyment of it may often be inferred by the child's reaction to and persistence with certain activities. The skillful therapist who is a diligent observer can usually identify favored activities in even the most severely involved child.

Typically, practicing occupational therapists perform this type of analysis in their head. **Figure 3-5** briefly lists the steps therapists perform to complete client-focused activity analyses, and **Figure 3-6** lists some of the aspects of the activity and the client that therapists must consider. As we discuss in Chapters Five and Six, generally this process is guided by a particular frame of reference or multiple frames of reference. Often, this process occurs quickly during a session with a client and allows the therapist to rapidly make adjustments in the activity or to rapidly select an alternative activity to allow the client success.

■ PLAY ASSESSMENT AS A BASELINE FOR GOAL WRITING

Previously (see Table 3-1, Figure 3-1, and Figure 3-2), we highlighted a variety of measures to assist in answering the "w" questions of play for pediatric clients. For any one child, multiple methods will likely be used to gather the information you need. However, we have emphasized the importance of activity analysis as a primary method of ongoing assessment with the pediatric client during play.

The importance of the formal evaluation of play is that it may lead us to a greater emphasis on play as a worthwhile outcome of our intervention and to the inclusion of specific goals for play. The outcome of the evaluation process, if therapy is to be initiated, is that occupational therapists must write goals to guide intervention and measure effectiveness. Although there are many "how to" guides for writing measurable goals and objectives, there is limited information available to help pediatric therapists write goals and objectives for play.

If we as occupational therapists value play as an occupation, play should be an explicit goal of occupational therapy (Bundy, 1993). A playful approach is most likely to be used in intervention when the goals are to build playfulness or to build play skills. Therapists may not be accustomed to writing play goals and objectives, but we recommend that they become a commonly included goal area when needed. Examples of goals in the realm of play and playfulness may be to self-initiate play, maintain independent play, engage in social play, or participate in a variety of play activities. Goals may also target general or specific play skills. **Figure 3-7** provides examples that may help you to begin to write goals and objectives in this area.

Figure 3-4   Steps to Completing a General Activity Analysis

1. Perform the activity oneself and consider the assumptions and associations that the activity brings to mind. For example, bike riding may be associated with fear in someone who was never good at it as a child, or dread in someone who was always left out when his or her friends went bike riding. In contrast, bike riding may surface pleasant memories of enjoyable summer days spent with lots of neighborhood friends. Bike riding is an activity that does not have specific childhood connotations because many adults also ride bikes. However, there is a developmental component to this activity in that very young children either do this activity differently or not at all because they are not developmentally ready.

2. Observe another person or multiple people completing the same activity. For example, view the videos provided of children riding bikes. What do you see emerge as the constants of this activity? How do the children differ in their performance from each other and from you?

3. Begin the activity analysis by naming and describing the activity. For example, bike riding: an activity using a two- or three-wheeled nonmotorized piece of equipment that moves through space by rolling, with the energy for movement provided by an individual's propulsion with either arms or legs.

4. List all steps and actions required of the activity and note variations in the order of steps when different people do the same activity. It may be important to consider step 2 to assist in this step. See the example of the general activity analysis provided in Appendix 3-2.

5. List all equipment and materials needed for the activity.

6. Describe the space needed for the activity and variations possible.

7. Describe the social demands and opportunities of the activity.

8. List any precautions or safety issues for completing this activity.

9. Describe the possible gender, cultural, or social biases related to this activity.

10. Describe the expected outcome of the activity and any possible variations.

11. Describe the required client factors, performance components, and performance skills required of this activity, as well as the sensory inputs provided by the activity.

Compiled from multiple sources listed in text

Figure 3-5   Steps to Completing Client-Focused Activity Analyses

1. The therapist observes a client completing an activity by watching the performance of each individual step.

2. The therapist considers which frame of reference is appropriate to use based on what is known about the client through evaluation.

3. The therapist observes specific features of activity performance based upon the frame(s) of reference chosen.

4. The therapist notes client's difficulty and hypothesizes the possible cause(s).

5. The therapist compares what is required by the task (what is known about the activity from general activity analysis) with the client's skills, abilities, likes, and dislikes gathered from the evaluation process to note discrepancies that could be removed or diminished through careful grading or adaptation, and ways to improve the meaningfulness of the activity for the child.

Compiled from multiple sources listed in text

Figure 3-6   Therapist Considerations During Client-Focused Activity Analysis

- What does this child like, enjoy, prefer?
- What motivates this child to perform? (intrinsic or extrinsic motivations; praise, high-fives, treats, choice of preferred activity, own personal challenge, competition with others, adult reactions)
- What memories might this child have in regard to this activity?
- Has the child had past success or failure with this activity or a similar activity?
- How does the child's family feel about this activity?
- Do the child's friends or siblings participate in this activity?
- How is the child's frustration tolerance?
- Is the child afraid of this activity or similar activities?
- What about this context supports or hinders the child's performance?
- Might the child be more willing to participate in an altered context (for example, more or less observation by peers, more or less competition with others, parent watching or not, different size room, room with different sensory features—quieter/louder, dimmer/brighter)

Compiled from multiple sources listed in text

Figure 3-7   Examples of General Play Goals

- Play with a variety of _____ [objects, toys, partners, themes, etc.]
- Increase diversity/variety, complexity, and creativity of play
- Engage playfully with persons or objects
- Participate in active physical/challenging play
- Sustain play to achieve mastery
- Express success in play
- Participate in _____ [type] game
- Participate in play in _____ [social, physical, or temporal] context
- Transition from one activity to another
- Improve motivation to play
- Initiate play activity of own choice
- Participate in social/peer play (e.g., parallel, interactive)
- Wait for playmate's response/turn
- Express choices/desires/wants with peer
- Use object or toy in novel/functional/symbolic way
- Enter into an activity with playmates without disrupting the play process
- Pretend to be a "character"

Based on ideas from Baranek, Reinhartsen, & Wannamaker (2001), Florey & Greene (2008), Miller & Kuhaneck (2008), and Miller & Miller-Kuhaneck (2008)

■ CONCLUSION

The examination of play as an occupation, considering its form, function, and meaning, is an important part of pediatric occupational therapy practice. The evaluation of play can be accomplished through the use of formal assessment tools, as well as interviews of the child and caregiver and naturalistic observation. Activity analysis should play a crucial role in understanding the activity characteristics of preferred activities and the proper activity–child match.

In our review of the history, purpose, and process of activity analysis, we stressed the importance of activity analysis to our profession. We described how a process initially used to examine motion for efficiency in labor eventually became a staple of occupational therapy practice, allowing us to select and adapt activities carefully for a variety of clients with highly individual needs. We delineated two specific types of activity analysis and described the process of each. In our practice with pediatric clients, we believe that skill in both forms of activity analysis is essential for the practitioner to use the occupation of play artfully in intervention. We invite the student, novice therapist, and experienced therapist alike to practice the skill of general activity analysis and to apply the skill of client-focused activity analysis creatively to their intervention with pediatric clients, as we do in Section Three of this book. Next, we turn to another essential skill for the pediatric occupational therapist: therapeutic use of self.

Appendix 3-1

General Activity Analysis Format with Explanations

Name of Activity:

Description of Activity:

Global Demands of the Activity: (Does the activity require physical strength, exceptional memory, precise coordination? When you think of this activity, what appears to be the primary requirement for it?)

Assumptions About This Activity and Associations Regarding This Activity: (For what age group is this activity appropriate? Is it typically associated with either gender? Does this activity have potential positive or negative connotations for someone? Are there cultural associations?)

Materials Needed for Activity: (List all equipment, tools, and supplies needed. Are there monetary costs involved?)

Space Requirements for This Activity: (Large vs. small space, quiet space, open space, cluttered space, well-lit space, darkened space, etc.)

Time Requirements for This Activity: (How long does it take to complete? Can it be broken up into smaller parts and completed over successive sessions? Do any of the steps require a specific period of time?)

Safety Precautions for This Activity: (Is there a potential for physical harm, allergic reaction, psychological distress, dust, fumes, skin irritations, poisons, injury with tools?)

List all steps for this activity.

Step One _____

Step Two _____

Step Three _____

Step Four _____

Step Five _____

(Add lines as needed)

For each of the previously listed steps, fill out this grid.
(You will have multiple copies of this grid as you analyze each step of the activity in a very detailed fashion.)

Step # _____	List step here
Sensory input/feedback provided (Visual, auditory, olfactory, gustatory, proprioceptive, vestibular, touch/pain/temperature)	
Motor output required (Specify the motion and the coordination needed—accuracy and smoothness)	
Specific muscles and joints used and range of motion required	
Laterality and crossing midline required (Bilateral or unilateral/symmetrical or asymmetrical/reciprocal)	
Strength required (Does gravity assist or hinder? Is the motion resisted?)	
Endurance required (How many repetitions are needed?)	
Position/posture required	
Body awareness required	
Mobility required	
Novelty of the motion/amount of praxis required	

Cognitive Requirements of This Activity: How much does one need a good attention span and strong concentration? What are the memory requirements of this activity? How much monitoring is required while completing the activity? How much planning is required? What is the nature of problem solving required to this activity? Is logic required? Must one be fully oriented to person, place, and time? What level of arousal is required? How much independent choice making is required? Does one need good judgment for this activity? Is safety awareness an issue? Does the activity require symbolic or abstract thinking? Does the activity require categorization? How much new learning is required? How much sequencing is required?

Perceptual Requirements of This Activity: Does this activity require one to be able to identify or match by color, size, shape/form? Must one know right from left? Is figure-ground perception required? Is depth perception required? How much visual-perceptual-motor integration is required? Does the activity require stereognosis? Is it important to have a good body scheme to be able to complete this activity?

Social-Emotional and Psychological Aspects of This Activity: Is this activity structured or unstructured? Does it have a predictable outcome or unpredictable outcome? How much creativity and expression is allowed? How much interaction is involved in this activity? How much choice is allowed? How much delay of gratification is needed? What motivating factors are there in this activity? How much does this activity provide a sense of control, a sense of productivity, a sense of competence, and a sense of achievement? How much does this activity allow interaction, cooperation, sharing, and conversation? How much does this activity allow creativity and individuality? How challenging is the activity, and how much opportunity is there for success? Can it be done alone, or does it require social interaction? Does it require sharing, taking turns, dealing with competition?

Appendix 3-2

Example of Completed Activity Analysis on Bike Riding

Name of activity: Bike riding

Description of Activity: An activity using a two- or three-wheeled nonmotorized piece of equipment that moves through space by rolling, with the energy for movement provided by an individual's propulsion with either arms or legs.

Global Demands of the Activity: Bike riding requires balance, endurance, and vision for safe maneuvering about the environment.

Assumptions About This Activity and Associations Regarding This Activity: Bike riding is appropriate for all individuals above the age of 3. Younger children may ride a tricycle or big wheel, whereas children slightly older may use training wheels until eventually, older children and adults can ride a two-wheeled bike. Elderly individuals may continue to ride bicycles if physically able and can also revert to adult tricycles if balance becomes a problem. Those with limited mobility of lower extremity can use bikes with hand pedals. Bike riding does not have strong gender connotations, and this activity is completed in many parts of the world. In the United States, it is primarily an activity of leisure, but in other cultures, bike riding is a primary mode of transportation and may be highly valued.

Materials Needed for Activity: An individual needs a bike, and bikes can vary in cost. For individuals serious about riding distances or racing, bikes can be quite costly. However, bikes can often be found secondhand as well, which can reduce costs. Helmets may be required as well. These vary in price but can be costly.

Space Requirements for This Activity: For biking, one needs an area that is large enough to allow for mobility through space. Typically, bikes are ridden outdoors, but one can use a bike stand to elevate the back tires and allow indoor riding for exercise. A bike can be ridden indoors in a large room without carpeting, such as a gymnasium.

Time Requirements for This Activity: Bike riding can be completed for as long or short a period as the individual desires. There is no specific time period required. However, for endurance building or exercise training, longer periods are required.

Safety Precautions for This Activity: There are significant safety issues with this activity. First, an individual could lose his or her balance and fall, injuring a variety of different body parts in the process. Second, if riding outdoors, and especially on the road, an individual could be injured by a motor vehicle. Helmets are required in many areas by law to prevent head injuries while biking. Adequate lighting is important for safety.

List all steps for this activity.

Step One With the bike leaning against a wall, pick up bike and grasp handlebars

Step Two Put one leg over bike, straddle seat

Step Three Sit on bike seat

Step Four Put one foot on one pedal

Step Five Lift other foot and begin to push pedal with the first foot

Step Six Alternate feet, pushing one pedal first, then the next

Step Seven Maintain handlebars in appropriate position to direct the bike to where you want to go, avoiding obstacles

Step #1	With bike leaning against a wall, pick up bike and grasp handlebars
Sensory input/feedback provided	Slight tactile input provided by grasp, proprioceptive input varies with the weight of the bike
Motor output required	Reach and grasp is required. Accurate reach to target is needed, although smoothness is not necessary
Specific muscles and joints used and range of motion required	Reach: elbow flexors and extensors, shoulder flexors and extensors Grasp: finger extensors and flexors, wrist extensors; no extreme range of motion is needed
Laterality and crossing midline required	Crossing midline is not required. Motion is either unilateral or bilateral. If bilateral, it will be symmetrical.
Strength required	The strength required depends on the weight of the bike, but from a leaning position, the strength required to lean the bike upright is not excessive. The motion is primarily in a horizontal plane; therefore, gravity neither helps nor hinders. If the bike is lying on the ground, gravity hinders the lifting of the bike.
Endurance required	Only one repetition of this step is needed. Minimal endurance is required.
Position/posture required	Although this step could be completed from a seated position, it is most often completed while standing.
Body awareness required	Minimal body awareness is required, although the child must get close enough to be able to reach and must not pull the bike so hard that it hits his or her body.
Mobility required	Minimal mobility is required for this step.
Novelty of the motion/amount of praxis required	Reach and grasp usually is an automatic motion for most children, not requiring significant praxis.

Step #2	Put one leg over bike, straddle seat
Sensory input/feedback provided	Tactile and visual cue of bike seat Slight vestibular input as posture changes to lift leg over bike.
Motor output required	Accuracy in raising leg high enough to clear seat Coordination and balance to stand on one foot while swinging leg over
Specific muscles and joints used and range of motion required	Hip flexors, knee flexors and extensors, hip abductors Significant range of motion is required in hip and knee to bend and swing leg over height of seat. Finger flexors to grasp handlebars

Laterality and crossing midline required	This is a unilateral asymmetrical action with one leg that does not require midline crossing. One leg stabilizes while the other moves. Arms are holding handlebars.
Strength required	This motion is against gravity. Sufficient strength against gravity to raise knee and hip over the seat and maintain standing on one leg is needed.
Endurance required	1 repetition, low demand on endurance
Position/posture required	Completed while standing, at times standing on one foot
Body awareness required	Significant body awareness to position self appropriately and judge height of leg swing
Mobility required	Balance and weight shift are required, no transitional movements
Novelty of the motion/amount of praxis required	Praxis required to plan and judge height and force of leg swing while maintaining balance; however, on familiar bike or for those familiar with bike riding, action may be more automatic
Step #3	Sit on bike seat
Sensory input/feedback provided	Tactile input from seat and handlebars
Motor output required	Accuracy to sit on seat Balance and coordination to hold bars and to maintain bike while sitting down
Specific muscles and joints used and range of motion required	Hip and knee flexors to sit Sufficient range of motion to sit depending on height of seat and bike
Laterality and crossing midline required	Symmetrical action, no midline crossing
Strength required	Gravity assists to lower to the seat
Endurance required	1 repetition, low endurance demand
Position/posture required	Seated posture on bike with seat supporting and hands on handlebars
Body awareness required	Minimal body awareness for this step
Mobility required	Minimal mobility for this step
Novelty of the motion/amount of praxis required	Minimal praxis, although accuracy needed if the seat is small

Step #4	Put one foot on one pedal
Sensory input/feedback provided	Tactile cue of pedal touching foot for locating pedal Proprioceptive input as bike leans
Motor output required	Accurate coordination of vision and tactile cue of pedal to place foot properly Balance to maintain oneself upright as one foot is lifted
Specific muscles and joints used and range of motion required	Hip and knee flexors, ankle dorsiflexors, adequate hip and knee flexion to lift leg to pedal
Laterality and crossing midline required	Unilateral action with one foot, no midline crossing
Strength required	Action against gravity, minimal strength against gravity to raise hip and knee
Endurance required	1 repetition, minimal demand
Position/posture required	Seated posture
Body awareness required	Minimal awareness to place foot with accuracy
Mobility required	Minimal demand on mobility
Novelty of the motion/amount of praxis required	Demand on praxis to plan and move foot to find pedal; pedal may not always be in same position

Step #5	Lift other foot and begin to push pedal with the first foot
Sensory input/feedback provided	Tactile cue of other pedal Proprioceptive feedback when pushing pedal Vestibular feedback for balancing bike
Motor output required	Coordination and smoothness to balance on bike while lifting the stabilizing foot Accuracy to reach to pedal quickly while maintaining balance Coordination of both feet to start pedaling
Specific muscles and joints used and range of motion required	Hip and knee flexors to reach pedal; adequate range of motion to reach pedal location Ankle plantar flexors to push pedal to move; minimal range of motion to push pedal
Laterality and crossing midline required	Unilateral movement of foot up to pedal Bilateral reciprocal movement to begin pedaling motion

Strength required	Gravity hinders when placing foot, then assists when pushing down pedal. Motion of pedal is also resisted by bike chain, type and texture of surface
Endurance required	1 repetition for this step; minimal demand
Position/posture required	Seated—balancing on bike seat
Body awareness required	Significant body awareness to maintain position of body on moving bike and balance
Mobility required	Lower body mobility as pedaling begins
Novelty of the motion/amount of praxis required	Praxis to coordinate movement to get pedaling going when skill is being learned. If familiar skill, this becomes automatic unless new bike, height of seat, etc., is introduced.

Step #6	Alternate feet, pushing one pedal first, then the next
Sensory input/feedback provided	Proprioceptive and tactile input of pedal and handlebars Vestibular input as bike moves Visual input as bike is directed
Motor output required	Bilateral coordination and smoothness of legs to pedal Coordination of arms steering while pedaling Balance
Specific muscles and joints used and range of motion required	Knee flexors and extensors and ankle plantar flexors and dorsiflexors Sufficient range of motion for full revolution of the pedals required, varies based on seat height
Laterality and crossing midline required	Bilateral reciprocal movement
Strength required	Gravity assists when pushing pedal down; however, motion resisted by bike chain and terrain Significant strength is required to bike uphill, minimal for downhill
Endurance required	Many repetitions, significant endurance demand
Position/posture required	Seated—balancing on bike seat
Body awareness required	Must maintain seated balance on moving bike
Mobility required	Lower body mobility
Novelty of the motion/amount of praxis required	With repetitions, actual pedaling does not place high demand on praxis

Step #7	Maintain handlebars in appropriate position to direct the bike to where you want to go, avoiding obstacles
Sensory input/feedback provided	Tactile and proprioceptive input from handlebars Visual input for direction Vestibular input as bike moves
Motor output required	Smoothness during steering, coordination for pedaling and steering at the same time Balance
Specific muscles and joints used and range of motion required	Shoulder flexors and extensors to steer bike Finger flexors to grip handlebars
Laterality and crossing midline required	Bilateral reciprocal movement for steering
Strength required	Motion is resisted by terrain and bike wheel/handlebars
Endurance required	Endurance to maintain grasp and multiple repetitions of turning or maintaining handlebars
Position/posture required	Seated—balancing on bike seat
Body awareness required	Significant awareness of maintaining balance on bike seat while leaning for turns or if bumps in terrain
Mobility required	Mobility demands remain the same
Novelty of the motion/amount of praxis required	Significant praxis involved to avoid obstacles and stay on course

Cognitive Requirements of This Activity: Bike riding requires significant attention to avoid obstacles and remain safe and significant continual monitoring of one's performance. Memory is required to know where one has ridden and how to get back to the beginning or to where one is supposed to go. Planning is required in terms of where to go, but once one has learned to ride, the process becomes somewhat automatic. Problem solving may only be necessary if one gets lost or something breaks (on the bike, for example). Choicemaking occurs primarily in the decisions regarding where to go and when (e.g., in deciding whether to cross the street). Significant judgment is needed for safety in terms of where to ride or not ride and when to start and stop.

Perceptual Requirements of This Activity: Bike riding requires the ability to visually discriminate a multitude of objects to avoid obstacles and not crash and be hurt. Visual abilities must also be strong for the eyes to maintain focus on objects while in motion and determine the speed of approach based on the visual cues provided by objects as they get nearer (depth perception is very important for this activity). One must know right and left to follow directions and not get lost while going somewhere, but this can be less important if following someone else. Color perception can be important if one is riding where traffic lights will need to be followed.

Social-Emotional and Psychological Aspects of This Activity: Bike riding can be a very unstructured activity or very structured if one is training for some race or event. Typically, children bike ride with friends or family in an unstructured way, although this activity can be done alone. There may or may not be a destination in mind. This is not a very creative activity, but significant choice can be allowed in where to go and which way to get there, as long as the roadways are safe. Generally, bike riding does not require much in the way of sharing or taking turns unless riding in single file and taking turns being in front. There can be peer interaction if riding with friends in the neighborhood or on a bike path. Bike riding can be very motivating as a peer activity, and the ability of a child to learn to ride without training wheels can either bolster or dampen self-esteem and feelings of competence at certain ages (typically about 5). Bike riding can provide significant feelings of independence and control in older children who are allowed the freedom to leave the home area and roam somewhat freely.

Bike riding is a very challenging activity that can be very difficult to learn and may lead to frustration and anger. A child needs good frustration tolerance and patience while learning this activity. Additionally, while learning to ride without training wheels, there may be significant fear and anxiety. A fall early in the process may add to fear and anxiety.

For those who desire greater challenge, individuals could explore professional or amateur bicycle racing, motor cross with jumps, and other competitive bicycle events. Individuals may also want to learn bicycle maintenance or building from parts.

4

Being Playful: Therapeutic Use of Self in Pediatric Occupational Therapy

After reading this chapter the reader will

1. Define therapeutic use of self and explain core components.

2. Communicate the value of a playful therapeutic use of self for pediatric clients, caregivers, and therapists.

3. Describe and apply strategies for therapeutic use of self to communicate playfully with a pediatric client.

4. Describe precautions and practical considerations for matching strategies for therapeutic use of self to the individual child's developmental level.

5. Explain how empathy and rapport promote a playful intervention environment.

6. Discuss issues regarding awareness and management of the therapist's own needs, attitudes, and roles in pediatric occupational therapy.

> *Whoever wants to understand much must play much.*
> —Gottfried Benn

As discussed in Chapter Two, occupational therapists believe that play is a primary occupation of children and is essential to client-centered pediatric occupational therapy practice. Play is both a part of and an outcome of occupational therapy. Playful occupational therapy sessions encourage clients to be active participants and to participate in the valued occupation of play.

Playful occupational therapy sessions start with the personal dynamics of the child and the occupational therapist. If the child has a strong sense of playfulness and a predisposition to play, then the occupational therapist need make few adaptations in her or his demeanor for that

client. If, however, as is more likely the case, the child's playfulness is restricted in some way, the occupational therapist must take the professional responsibility for creating a playful environment. The child's own playfulness may be limited. Or, the therapeutic activities that address our clients' needs often are, by their nature, more effortful than playful.

Therapy is often at odds with play (Hellendoorn, 1994). In these less playful situations, the occupational therapist uses activity analysis to shape play activities and therapeutic use of self to promote an environment where the child can approach the activities as play. The occupational therapist draws on therapeutic use of self to communicate to the child that therapy can be fun and to develop a shared playful therapeutic relationship to enable the child's individual playfulness to emerge. This artful aspect of practice is refined through methodical self-reflection. This chapter illustrates this process of playful therapeutic use of self, its core components, and its importance to satisfying and effective pediatric occupational therapy.

■ THERAPEUTIC USE OF SELF: AN ARTFUL TOOL OF PRACTICE

When an occupational therapist consciously "use[s] his or her personality, insights, perceptions, and judgments as part of the therapeutic process," this is known as therapeutic use of self (American Occupational Therapy Association, 2008, p. 653). As an occupational therapist engages in therapeutic use of self, he or she becomes a *tool* of practice (Mosey, 1986). Every response and interaction is potentially therapeutic if the occupational therapist makes a conscious effort to act in a way that best meets the client's needs and facilitates the therapeutic process. Mosey (1986) explained that therapeutic use of self "involves a planned interaction with another person in order to alleviate fear or anxiety, provide reassurance, obtain necessary information, provide information, give advice, and assist the other individual to gain more appreciation of, more expression of, and more functional use of his or her latent inner resources" (p. 199).

Therapeutic use of self is an artful aspect of practice that involves a high level of creative interaction with individual clients (Mosey, 1981; Peloquin, 1990; Price, 2009). This is not the romantic, idealized view of creativity as simple intrinsic ability, because that notion overlooks the disciplined work and problem solving actually involved in creativity (Sapp, 1995). Whereas natural talents and abilities are certainly helpful, the use of problem solving, the ability to generate and integrate new ideas, and the discipline to apply knowledge, all of which are critical to creativity, must be learned and cultivated (Feldhusen & Goh, 1995; Sapp, 1995).

Everyone has the potential to be creative (Runco, 2007; Sternberg, 2006). Creativity is an intentional choice a person makes, a potential fulfilled by choosing to exercise it in everyday activities through mindful and creative actions rather than assumptions and routine actions (Runco, 2007). Creativity is an intrinsic part of the philosophy of occupational therapy (Schmid, 2004) and is especially linked to play and spirituality in occupational therapy (Toomey, 2003). Blanche (1992) urged occupational therapists to develop creativity to better meet the challenges of practice. Suggestions for enhancing creativity in occupational therapy are provided in **Table 4-1.**

The form of therapeutic use of self varies dramatically between clients and at different points in time with the same client (Peloquin, 1990; Price, 2009; Taylor, 2008). The occupational therapist must respond to the individualized needs of a client at that particular point in time. Therefore, the occupational therapist must be very sensitive to the client's feelings and needs with a view toward future therapeutic goals (Mosey, 1981, 1986). The occupational therapist must exercise a high degree of self-control to manage his or her feelings, needs, and values to refrain from responding spontaneously. Additionally, the occupational therapist must resist the external pressures to use only routine, standardized protocols and instead attend to the individual client's needs and interactions (Hinojosa, 2007). This conscious approach is enacted in a relaxed, informal manner for the client (Mosey, 1986; Palmadottir, 2006). A therapeutic use of self requires analytical forethought

and careful clinical reasoning to determine a response that matches the client's therapeutic needs (Mosey, 1981, 1986). Communication, empathy, rapport, and reflective self-awareness are key components and are discussed in more detail in the following sections.

Communication

Communication, both verbal and nonverbal, is part of therapeutic use of self (Mosey, 1981, 1986; Punwar, 2000; Schwartzberg, 1993) and is essential to establishing a playful environment. For treatment activities to be experienced as play, they must be marked by the therapist and child as play and as distinctly different from work or other

Table 4-1   Methods for Enhancing Creativity in Occupational Therapy

- Change physical location to give new perspective
- Redefine the problem
- Simplify complex situations into a core problem/issue
- Consider the broader, bigger problem
- Consider slight alternatives and variations to a problem
- Find or apply an analogy of how this situation is similar to something else you know about
- Consider similarities/analogies in nature
- Borrow or adapt other similar approaches from others (e.g., from this book, from other occupational therapists)
- Experiment with different ideas
- Question assumptions
- Consider an approach that is contrary to conventionally accepted ideas
- Find ways to change restrictive rules or the environment to allow other options
- Keep an open mind
- Entertain multiple possibilities (no one right answer)
- Be persistent, because effort is required for creativity to emerge
- Believe in your creative potential

Adapted from Blanche (1992) and Runco (2007)

activities (Bateson, 1972; Skard & Bundy, 2008; Henricks, 1999). This is quite similar to the typical process described in Chapter One, where both animals and children send play signals to potential playmates. If they are going to play with children, adults must understand a child's signals about what he or she wants to play, and they must also send clear signals that they want to play with the child.

Understanding the Communication Signals of a Pediatric Client

Children do not possess the same language and communication skills as adults (Curtin, 2001; Graue & Walsh, 1995), and children with disabilities may have additional limitations in their communication abilities. Further complicating the therapist's attempts to understand the pediatric client are that children in general experience the world differently from adults because of differences in development and social position (Corsaro & Eder, 1990; Fine & Sandstrom, 1988; Glassner, 1976; Kaplan, 1997). Children with disabilities may have further sensory perceptual and motor differences that also change their experiences of the world (i.e., Durig, 1996; Frank, 2000; Goode, 1980; Grandin, 1995). Because of these differences between occupational therapists and their pediatric clients, understanding the child as an occupational being can be very challenging (Spitzer, 2003a, 2003b).

The occupational therapist must observe, listen, and interpret a child's cues to determine the child's interests and motivation (Holloway, 2008; Knox, 2008; Spitzer,

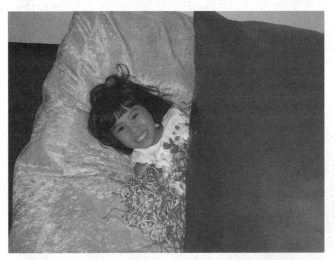

To develop empathy and rapport with a pediatric client, the occupational therapist strives to understand and identify the child's interests regarding what he or she likes and wants to do. Smiles, eye gaze, reaching, and turning toward an activity are common ways that children communicate their interests.

2003a). Possible nonverbal indicators of engagement and interest in an activity include increased self-initiated interaction, increased frequency and/or duration of eye contact, increased affect, increased attention span, increased participation, behavior modulation, and increased vocalizations and/or communication (Brown et al., 2008). Even children with significant speech and motor impairments can communicate preference for a toy or other material through orienting (noticing and looking or listening), affective responses (smiling, swinging arms, or verbalizations), and leaning toward a preferred object (Van Tubbergen, Warschausky, Birnholz, & Baker, 2008). Specific strategies for understanding the pediatric client's perspective are listed in **Table 4-2**.

When attempting to understand the child's perspective, the occupational therapist must operate "as if" the child provided intentional communication, assuming the child meant something by his or her actions. The occupational therapist must interpret and act as if the child's actions have meaning regardless of a judgment of the child actually conceptualizing and communicating that point. This is not an "objective" assessment of the child's skill level but a focus on the child's *potential* and attempts to become skilled. For example, the child might make a vocalization that sounds almost like a word. The adult often acts as if the child "talked" (Brazelton, Koslowski, & Main, 1974; Trevarthen, 1980). The adult takes the next step of relating a child's sounds to the most likely word or phrase and then reacts as if this was the word the child intended. For example, the child may say "ga-ooo" and the therapist may interpret this as "got you" and then initiate a "got you" game. The occupational therapist fills in the gaps and reacts as if the child did say that word, sometimes repeating that word, even if the therapist is surprised because the child has not said this word before, or it seems like a leap beyond previously seen skills and abilities. Many children do not develop in a step-by-step linear fashion. If the therapist incorporates what he or she thought the child "said," the therapist must still allow the child the opportunity to accept or reject this new word. In another case, the child might look at or reach in the direction of a toy, and the occupational therapist can offer to include the toy. Again, the occupational therapist must also be open to the child's reactions as to whether the child truly was interested in the toy. In this way, the occupational therapist is actively part of understanding and demonstrating this understanding of the child. It is a reciprocal, shared process of relating to each other. This is the foundation for a therapeutic relationship.

Table 4-2   Strategies to Enhance Understanding of Pediatric Clients

- Suspend adult assumptions (i.e., superiority) (Curtin, 2001; Fine & Sandstrom, 1988)
- Level power differences/inequality—avoid being an authority figure, minimize stopping and directing of the client (Curtin, 2001; Fine & Sandstrom, 1988)
- Look for effect/impact of adult presence (Fine & Sandstrom, 1988)
- Assume all actions are potentially communicative (Durig, 1996)
- Attend to communication through occupational engagement, especially shared occupations (Grandin & Scariano, 1986; Spitzer, 2003a; Williams, 1992)
- Look for individualized communication strategies around shared routines, physical environment, likes and dislikes, and bodily expressions (Goode, 1980, 1994; Spitzer, 2003a)
- Develop a shared history with the client—understand their favorite objects and preferences, and participate in activities with them (Goode, 1980, 1994; Spitzer, 2003a)
- Interview other people knowledgeable about the client
- Follow the client's directions—"passive obedience" (Goode, 1980)
- Imitate, physically simulate, or imagine the individual's sensory experience of the occupation to "feel" the experience (Goode, 1980; Spitzer 2003a)
- Sharpen conscious awareness of various auditory, visual, tactile, and kinesthetic sensations (Spitzer, 2003a)

From Spitzer (2004) chapter in *Autism: A Comprehensive Occupational Therapy Approach* (2nd ed., p. 89), which was adapted from original article published in the *American Journal of Occupational Therapy* (Spitzer, 2003, p. 71). Copyright 2004 by the American Occupational Therapy Association. Reproduced with permission of American Occupational Therapy Association via Copyright Clearance Center.

When the occupational therapist uses this information to develop individually tailored activities and approaches, the pediatric client will begin to feel understood (Mattingly & Fleming, 1994; Price & Miner, 2007). The same physical materials used with similar motor actions can become dramatically different play activities. For example, one child interested in construction might be offered fuzzy balls to pick up with tongs like a crane, whereas another child might be offered the same materials as special eating tools in an outer-space diner (see Chapter Six for details on how to create individualized therapeutic play activities). These personal, individualized procedures demonstrate the occupational therapists' knowledge of the client. This communication is the beginning of developing empathy and rapport in the therapeutic relationship.

"This Is Fun!": Sending a Message of Play Through Nonverbal and Verbal Communication

The occupational therapist can mark therapy as play by sending a message that therapy is fun (Parham, 1992). This is not an automatic process because the mere presence of adults can predispose children to view activities as more work than play (Howard, Jenvey, & Hill, 2006). Playfulness is communicated through therapeutic use of self, whereby occupational therapists create a playful environment with verbal and nonverbal strategies as well as model playful engagement that the child may imitate. This is a graded process individualized to the child's own cognitive, social, and self-regulatory abilities. When matched to the child, this message of play helps the child *anticipate* and expect that the activity will be fun. This playful approach helps transform the activity into play.

In general, occupational therapists interact with clients through their physical orientation and voice characteristics (Langthaler, 1990, as cited by Mattingly & Fleming, 1994). Langthaler's research found that physical orientation consists of proxemics (body space/closeness), body orientation, gestures, head movements, eye movements, and facial expression. Touch may also be used (Mosey, 1981; Taylor, 2008). Occupational therapists carefully control their own behavior to convey an effective message to their clients (Mattingly & Fleming, 1994; Mosey, 1981).

Applying these strategies in pediatrics requires special consideration of how adults send playful communication signals that can be understood by clients of differing developmental abilities. Because most of the research on adult play communication with children comes from parent–child play studies, this research is reviewed and integrated

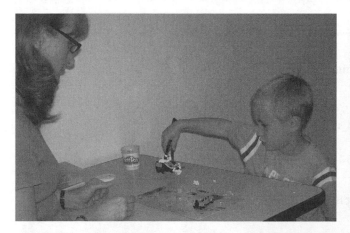
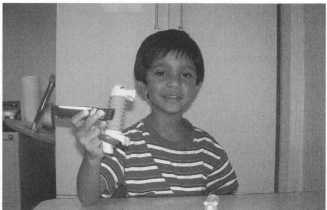

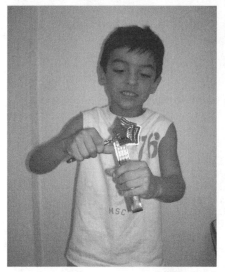
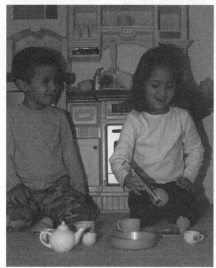
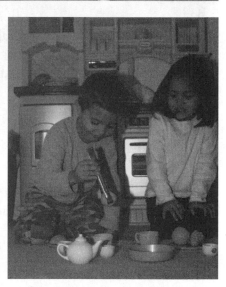

The occupational therapist demonstrates empathy and rapport with clients through personal, individualized procedures where the same materials can be used in different ways based on the child's individual interests and goals. Tongs can be used as a "crane" to pick up vehicles, as a way to transport animals to food, as a "weapon," or as a utensil for "eating" depending on the individual child.

with occupational therapy literature. Together this information provides rich details on specific strategies that occupational therapists can use with their pediatric clients to communicate that occupational therapy is play (**Table 4-3** and **Appendix 4-1**[1]). With infants, play is marked by the adult, parent, or therapist giving visual, auditory, and physical stimuli to the child. As the child develops, the play is more cooperative and collaborative, with the child taking an increasingly more active role. Both verbal and nonverbal communication is involved.

It is important to note that the amount of communication must be carefully balanced by the adult so that the child can maintain an arousal state that enables continued engagement in play (Parham, 1992; Power, 2000). Although a certain level of excitement and enthusiasm often

accompanies play, too much stimulation, even of a positive sort, can overload a child into a state of disorganization. This is usually a bigger concern in typically developing children during infancy (Power, 2000), but self-regulation difficulties may continue throughout childhood in children with disabilities. Adults must be sensitive to a child's need to withdraw, partially or completely, at times after a period of engagement (Brazelton et al., 1974; Brazelton & Tronick, 1980).

Nonverbal Communication. Adult nonverbal communication that initiates and sustains play includes eye gaze, facial expressions, and body language/movements (Power, 2000). Such nonverbal communication usually occurs in close but comfortable proximity (Hall, 1966/1982). If the adult is too far away, the child is less likely to notice these subtle actions in the distance.

---

[1] The appendices in this chapter are also available online at *www.jbpub.com.*

Table 4-3   Strategies to Communicate Playfulness

Therapist Sources of Communication	Specific Strategies/Techniques
Eyes	• Look at the child • Look between the child and a potential toy/play object
Face	• Exaggerate and hold positive emotional expressions, especially surprise, smiles, and concern • Imitate the child's expression
Body	• Turn toward the child • Exaggerate and slow body movements such as imitation, head nodding, head wagging, or head cocking • Hold out, manipulate, hide, or point to toys/objects
Touch	• Use touch as appropriate for the context to get attention and show something
Voice (vocalizations)	• Use a playful tone • Vary pitch, loudness, rhythm • Repeat sounds • Imitate sounds and ways that sounds are used by child
Language	• Imitate child's words • Match language to child's development • Use language in song, melody, rhythm, or different voice (e.g., accent) • Use "kid play" words, phrases, and sounds • Use humor, jokes, and mischievous tone • Talk as if toys or body parts were alive and thinking

Gaze. In newborns, the adult looks at the child extensively and usually initiates the gaze (Messer & Vietze, 1984). The child is more likely to look at the adult if the adult is looking at the child (Messer & Vietze, 1984), and playful interactions are more likely to occur when the adult is looking at the child (Stern, 1974). This adult gaze at a child is almost continuous, in violation of adult Western cultural standards for a more intermittent pattern (Stern, 1974). As the child develops, the adult may also look back and forth between the child and a potential play object/toy (Findji, 1993; Friedman et al., 1976). Similarly, the occupational therapist's eye gaze can communicate that the therapist is ready and open to play. However, the occupational therapist must also be cautious because some

individual children can tolerate only limited amounts of stimulation from eye gaze and may not look much at the therapist directly (Miller, 1996).

Facial Expressions. Adult facial expressions that initiate or sustain play include mock surprise, smiling, and concern/sympathy (Power, 2000; Stern, 1974). As the child begins to demonstrate clear facial expressions, the adult may also imitate the child's expressions to continue play. Mostly, the adult's facial expressions are positive. They also tend to be significantly more exaggerated and maintained for a longer time period than facial expressions used in adult communication. Exaggerated expressions communicate that the activity is fun in such a clear way that the child is more likely to register the message and respond in play. For the occupational therapist, holding positive exaggerated facial expressions can promote a playful environment (Parham, 1992).

Body Language. The adult's body movements that encourage play in children include imitating the child's hand and body movements; moving the head, such as nodding up and down, wagging side to side, and head cocking; facing and leaning toward the child; and holding out, manipulating, hiding, or pointing to toys/objects (Pawlby, 1977; Stern, 1974). Again, these actions tend to be exaggerated and slowed down in comparison with adult communication. Similar body language can be used by the occupational therapist to show that he or she is involved with the child's interests.

Touch. Pediatric occupational therapists rate therapeutic touch as important to their practice (Cole & McLean, 2003). Touch is used heavily in interactions with infants (Moszkowski & Stack, 2007)—tickling, crawling fingers up and down arms and legs, starting and stopping a light tap, and physically assisted games. As children get older, similar types of touch remain communicative but tend to decrease in frequency. Touch games are very playful. Tickling games often involve joyous laughter in humans and appear to have a biological basis that may be shared with other species (Panksepp & Burgdorf, 2003). Many

play themes such as play fighting or peek-a-boo may include touch. Even a tap to show an object or direct attention may be very effective to remind a child what to do or how to do something without explicitly directing him or her or breaking up the flow of play.

Sometimes therapists are uncomfortable with using touch to communicate because, among adults, touch tends to have connotations of affection, intimacy, and even sexuality (Aldis, 1975; Taylor, 2008). When done in a conscious way, however, it can be an effective therapeutic strategy. In some settings, touch is not allowed or is devalued. Pediatric occupational therapists must use touch in a way that is both careful and respectful but also caring. It is safest to touch on the hand and arm and within the client's visual range, asking permission or giving notification when possible (Taylor, 2008). In some cases, pediatric occupational therapists may need to advocate institutional changes so that caring touch can be used with their clients.

Vocalizations and Verbal Communication. Occupational therapists can use sounds and words in a playful way while still addressing therapeutic outcomes (Parham, 1992). Vocalizations and language can be matched to the child's developmental level to communicate playfulness.

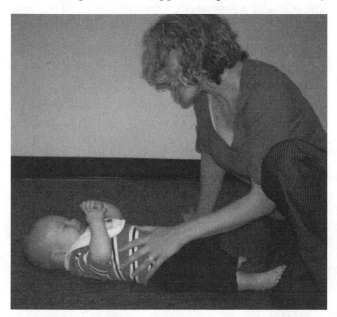

Playful communication with infants usually includes close proximity, eye gaze, and touch.

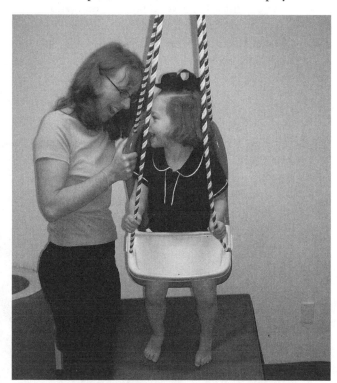

The occupational therapist communicates an openness and willingness to play by looking at, turning toward, getting close to, and smiling at the child.

Minimizing directive language takes a creative approach. Adults often use language to direct children to do things, a less-than-playful use of language. In fact, Shine and Acosta (1999) noted that play was usually ended by adult directions of how to behave, to clean up, or to explore a concept, or explanations. If the session is going to be playful, the occupational therapist generally must avoid using language to "direct" or "teach." Obviously, this is difficult, because we often need to direct or guide our clients to promote therapeutic outcomes. We may need to give them feedback about their performance, encourage them to try or persist in a challenging task, or change how they are doing the activity. Using alternative words and sounds and a light tone can shift the session to being more fun and less serious. Given that many children with disabilities also have deficits in auditory or language processing, additional modifications in selecting and using language may be needed.

Sounds. As children develop, adult and child communication in play tends to become increasingly verbal (Power, 2000). Initially, with infants, voice is used without much language. The adult uses vocal sounds to communicate playfulness. The ranges of pitch and loudness are broader than the ranges typically used in adult conversation (Power, 2000). These communicative sounds are marked by sudden changes in pitch, rhythm, and stress, and elongated vowel sounds (Aldis, 1975; Stern, 1974). Sounds and nonsense words may be repeated frequently (Aldis, 1975). At times, the adult's vocalizations may sound similar to features the child uses (Pawlby, 1977).

Words. As the child develops and interacts more with the adult, the adult tends to use more language. The adult commonly asks questions, praises the child, imitates the child's "words," and gives words to the child's utterances and actions (Halliday & Leslie, 1986; Shine & Acosta, 1999). Language becomes increasingly more complex and collaborative as the adult initiates, prompts, structures, and provides ideas to expand play, especially pretend play (Damast, Tamis-LeMonda, & Bornstein, 1996; Dunn, Wooding, & Hermann, 1977). Adult language is usually at a developmental level equal to or slightly higher than the child's development (Damast et al., 1996).

Because children with disabilities may have difficulty understanding language, the occupational therapist must use words selectively and monitor to ensure that the child understood what was said. Pairing words with clear and consistent intonation and body language provides a message that the child is more likely to understand. At times,

the occupational therapist will need to limit talking to avoid disrupting the child's focused engagement in the flow of play (Parham, 1992).

Same Words, Different Way. Any directive sounds more playful when said in an unconventional way, such as singing directions, repeating key words in a melodic rhythm, or using a voice different from one's normal speech pattern. In this way, the occupational therapist's use of speech is more like the way children themselves play with the sounds of language (Nilsen & Nilsen, 1978). Consider an occupational therapist who wants a child to work on fastening buttons and zippers. The occupational therapist can announce, "come sit down and do your buttons," "it is time for buttons and zippers," or "let's do buttons and zippers." Despite differing levels of directiveness, all these announcements send a similar message about an effortful activity on which the child needs to "work." But it can be transformed when the therapist sings these same words to a common children's song like "The Farmer in the Dell" (that is, punctuated with "Hi-ho the-dairy-oh"). Emphasizing particularly fun sounds and repeating the sounds in a rhythm can also change the way the child views this direction. For example, the occupational therapist can alter speed between slow and fast in saying, "it's time for button-zzzzz and zzz-ipper-zzzzz, and zzz-ipper-zzzzz and button-zzzzz. Button-zzzzz and zzz-ipper-zzzzz, and zzz-ipper-zzzzz and button-zzzzz." The activity can also become more playful by announcing in a slow robotic accent: "It is time for bu-ttons and zi-pper-s." The direction becomes so fun that children often like to repeat these phrases themselves in similar and modified ways, and sometimes even as they do the transformed work, as a self-talk strategy. For some children, the sounds themselves become reinforcing, and getting to hear the sound becomes a motivating reason to do an activity.

Kid Play Words and Sound Effects. Utilizing words and sounds that children commonly use provides feedback that facilitates a playful process in therapy, where the focus is on participation. This differs from serious, realistic, grown-up words that remind the child that he or she is working on something for which the quality of the performance is important. When mistakes happen, words and sound effects like "bonk," "oops," "oops-a-daisy," "ut-oh," or "ut-oh spaghetti-o-s" sound fun, helping to incorporate errors into play rather than stopping play to focus on the error. When the child misbehaves, words like "Hey silly goose, let's _____!" keep the session playful, rather than stopping to chastise the child or insisting on compliance (e.g., "no, come here.")

Positive feedback can also be incorporated into play. Standard adult comments of "good job" or "good work" reinforce that the adult is there to monitor and judge the quality of the child's performance. Words like "yeah," "wow," "yahoo," "zoom," "incredible," and "amazing" provide positive feedback in a way that maintains the flow of the play experience.

Children are often most interested in words that adults have been socialized not to use, such as "poop." Because they are seldom used, children find the words' novelty and adult reactions to be funny. If an occupational therapist wants to be playful, he or she may decide to go against adult social taboos and use these words in therapeutic ways. An example with Jacob[2] follows:

Jacob and Word Play

Jacob was fascinated with the word "poop." He loved to say "poop" and loved to watch adults get upset when he said it. He used this as a strategy to avoid and escape adult demands because it distracted adults from the activity at hand. His occupational therapist wanted to incorporate his love of the word "poop" into therapy sessions. After the occupational therapist explained her reasoning to Jacob's mother, she agreed. The occupational therapist began to incorporate the word "poop" into every activity such as drawing pictures of poop, tracing and writing the word poop, playing obstacle course games with brown bean-bag poop, and "Simon Says _____, poop." After four sessions, Jacob became tired of the word and wanted to play new games that no longer included the word "poop."

Learning Activity

Consider the case of Jacob:

- Are you comfortable with the occupational therapist's approach? Why or why not?
- How else could you communicate playfulness in working with Jacob?
- If Jacob's family culture was different, with strong values about appropriate behavior, and they did not want Jacob to talk about poop, what would you do differently?

---

[2]To protect confidentiality, all names and identifying information used throughout this book have been changed, except when specifically requested to use the real name.

Kidding Around. Adding humor (Vergeer & MacRae, 1993), jokes, and mischievousness can help build therapeutic relationships and lighten up otherwise serious work. Even work elements can be overly exaggerated to be playful elements. For example, the occupational therapist may present a challenge with mock concern or mischievousness, such as, "This is pretty tricky. Hmmm, do you think you can do this? Oh, no, this is too hard. What if you fall? I don't know if you can do it." A therapist might "conspire" with a child to scare or surprise mommy. Even when a child tries to avoid a challenge, the atmosphere can be kept playful by a mock chastisement of something like "Hey, no cheating-g-g-g." The laughter that follows can build attachment bonds among client, therapist, and others involved (Nelson, 2008).

Because humor involves a more complicated understanding of real and pretense, the occupational therapist must exercise caution in making sure that the level of humor is appropriate for the child's development. If not, children may misunderstand and believe they are being made fun-of (laughed at) or teased, an obviously unintended outcome. In the simplest sense, a child can find something humorous if he or she recognizes both that something is being said or done that is "wrong" and that it is *intentionally* done incorrectly. For example, putting a spoon on one's head when the person knows that a spoon is for eating is humorous if knowingly and intentionally done but is a mistake if done during meal time when trying to eat. The impossibility of the idea "Why don't you jump *under* the ball?" can be very funny for a 6-year-old who understands such language. Sometimes mistakes can have unintended funny consequences, such as tossing an eraser to a child and it lands in a nearby cup of water. When the therapist laughs at him- or herself or allows him- or herself to look silly, the therapist communicates a commitment to playfulness and an acceptance of his or her own shortcomings.

Clear, simple forms of joking actions accompanied by laughter can be at least understood by toddlers at 19 months of age and require less cognitive understanding than pretend play (Hoicka & Gattis, 2008). As children develop, they understand more subtle and ambiguous forms of humor. A sense of humor may be less present in the play of children with intellectual disabilities (Messier, Ferland, & Majnemer, 2008) or may take a different form. Because cognitive development can be difficult to assess in some children with disabilities, it is usually best to follow the child's lead in using humor. When the child laughs, this provides a good example of the type of humor the occupational therapist may use. But some children do not spontaneously laugh on their own. Clear, simple jokes of doing or saying what the child clearly knows "should not be" and smiling or laughing is usually a good way to introduce humor when there are concerns about cognitive understanding. Children's joke books and websites[3] can be good sources of ideas as well.

Personification. Children commonly use words to respond to and address inanimate objects, acting as if they are alive. They talk to a toy like it is a person who might do what they say or answer them (e.g., "good night toys" as the toys are put away, or "dollie wants to play _____"). Although this can have an element of pretend play, it is also different from pretend play. Or, it can be a particular type of humor if the child sees it as funny or comical.

An occupational therapist can use language in this alternate way to create more of a playful mode, especially for otherwise serious challenges. For example, Baron (1991) described using a client's favorite toy, a Pee Wee Herman figure, in occupational therapy to help with power struggles in a child with oppositional defiant disorder. Limit-setting and feedback were given to the child by Pee Wee Herman via the therapist's voice. The child accepted this input because he could pretend it "came from" his favorite toy instead of the adult authority figure.

The occupational therapist can also use this strategy without toys. For example, the occupational therapist who is working on in-hand manipulation skills with a child often faces the challenge of the child compensating in various less-than-therapeutic ways. The child may try to use the other hand to help or may push the one hand against his or her body or the table to provide assistance with the tasks, thereby defeating the activity's therapeutic purpose. In this situation, the occupational therapist can simply direct the child not to do that or to do it this way. But it remains hard work for the child. Instead, the occupational therapist can use a similar directive oriented toward the child's hand: "It's not your turn, hand. Let that other hand have his turn," or "Hey, hand, get to work. No cheating. You know the rules." Suddenly even chastisement in a mock serious tone can become play. The child is no longer being chastised but can join the adult therapist in "chastising" his hand.

Such a strategy can also be used to make mistakes more playful and lighthearted. For example, if the child misses attempts to throw a ball or put an object into a container, the occupational therapist can begin a pseudo-conversation with the ball: "Ball, you need to behave. He was putting you inside. You need to listen and go inside. Be a good ball and do what you are told. We'll give you another chance." Again, such humorous behavior on the part of the occupational therapist marks this activity as playful. Furthermore, it frees the pediatric client to switch temporarily from the worker role into an empowered director of "others."

Child Feedback and Handling Miscommunication

Whenever two people communicate, there is always potential for miscommunication. You can be assured that miscommunication occurs in therapy as well (Taylor, 2008). It is important to be watchful and recognize when it does occur. This way, you can quickly repair any unintended problems and tension in a therapeutic way (Taylor, 2008), and resend the message so that it is more likely to be registered correctly.

To determine if the child received the intended message about play, the occupational therapist must read the child's cues and reactions. When a practitioner is playful, the child usually is agreeable to the therapeutic activity at hand (Terr et al., 2007). Some children provide clear feedback that they understand the message of play. They may begin to be more playful through laughing, smiling, pretending, or extending the therapist's play ideas. Or, the child may react negatively through affect, statements, agitation, resistance, or destructive actions, suggesting that the occupational therapist's attempts to communicate playfulness have not been accepted. Common strategies that young children use to show that they find something unpleasant (not playful) include actively withdrawing, pushing away, ignoring, and fussing/crying (Brazelton et al., 1974). Some children with disabilities may provide limited feedback for our actions (Brazelton & Tronick, 1980; Greenspan, & Wieder, 1997). Their bodies may limit their abilities to react, or they may process information in a slow or limited way. In the absence of clear signals, at times, the occupational therapist must determine the most successful strategies and persist with those strategies. If a child has misunderstood the communication, then the strategies need to be modified to match the individual child's needs.

Empathy and Rapport in a Playful Therapeutic Relationship

Empathy and rapport allow the occupational therapist to engage in play with the child. Empathy is a deep

---

[3]For example, *http://www.activityvillage.co.uk/kids_jokes.htm*

understanding and caring about the child as an occupational being. With empathy, the occupational therapist can demonstrate genuine respect for the child so that therapeutic rapport can emerge (Peloquin, 1995; Price, 2009; Schwartzberg, 1993). When the child and family feel confident and trust the occupational therapist, they can take on greater challenges and greater risks, and even confront the potential for failure (Price, 2009). The therapist's empathy and rapport allow the child and family to play (Ferland, 2005).

Empathy in Occupational Therapy

Empathy is an informed caring. Empathy is a way of knowing about another person that involves both thinking and feeling at the same time (Peloquin, 1995). It is a way of knowing the client as a person, not just a disability or diagnosis. Empathy is based on developing an understanding of the child and what is important to him or her (Fleming, 1994; Price, 2009; Schwartzberg, 1993; Yerxa, 1967) and what is very difficult or negative for the child (Frank, 1958; Taylor, 2008). The therapist understands and feels the fears, doubts, hopes, and desires of the child and family. By understanding the child and family, the occupational therapist is able to share their view and have a sense of what it is like to be them (Peloquin, 1995). Occupational therapists must recognize similarities and differences between themselves and their clients. Beyond clinical knowledge about general experiences, occupational therapists need to understand their clients' particular experiences and feelings. Understanding is based on accepting the client as an equal person (Crepeau, 1991). Occupational therapists use empathetic understanding to inform empathic behavior and create an empathic relationship (Gahnstrom-Strandqvist, Tham, Josephsson, & Borell, 2000).

The empathic occupational therapist cares about the child (Peloquin, 1995). Caring is part of the therapeutic process (Peloquin, 1990, 1993). Caring humanizes the science of therapy (Gilfoyle, 1980). Without caring, clients are depersonalized (Peloquin, 1990, 1993). This is not providing care *to* or taking care *of* but caring *for* clients (Gilfoyle, 1980). Mayeroff (1971, p. 1) defined caring as helping another person "grow and actualize" the self. Rather than simply saying we care, occupational therapists demonstrate we care by doing things for and with clients (Mattingly & Fleming, 1994). Occupational therapists care about a client's growth, development, function, and adaptation (Gilfoyle, 1980; Mosey, 1981, 1986). Occupational therapists help patients to care about themselves, what they can do, and what they might be able to do

(Devereaux, 1984; Gilfoyle, 1980). Sometimes a therapist naturally wants to care for a client on a personal basis, whereas at other times, a therapist does not have a natural connection with emotional caring. In these latter situations, Wright-St. Clair (2001) recommended that therapists focus on the general professional ideal and moral obligation to care for clients' well-being. This general focus on a philosophy of caring allows us to "ethically care" for individual clients for whom we might not otherwise naturally care (Wright-St. Clair, 2001).

Rapport in a Therapeutic Occupational Therapy Relationship

The therapeutic relationship is essential to client-centered occupational therapy (Hinojosa, 2007; Tickle-Degnen, 2002) and is highly valued by occupational therapists (Taylor, Lee, Kielhofner, & Ketkar, 2009). Based on a survey of 129 practicing occupational therapists, Cole and McLean (2003) defined a therapeutic relationship as "a trusting connection and rapport established between therapist and client through collaboration, communication, therapist empathy and mutual understanding and respect" (pp. 33–34). The therapeutic relationship is developed in stages (Lloyd & Maas, 1991; Price, 2009). This relationship helps clients envision a future of possibilities and is intertwined with the therapeutic process in occupational therapy (Price, 2009). Clients trust that their occupational therapist is competent and will help them achieve meaningful outcomes (Devereaux, 1984; Frank, 1958; Gahnstrom-Strandqvist et al., 2000; Guidetti & Tham, 2002).

Rapport is a working alliance or bond between the occupational therapist and client (Tickle-Degnen, 2002). Rapport is at the *core* of meaningful occupational therapy, where clients find meaning in their occupations (Peloquin, 1995). Occupational therapists use a variety of specific strategies to build rapport in a therapeutic relationship (**Table 4-4**) and actively involve clients by providing choices and engaging in joint problem solving (Gahnstrom-Strandqvist et al., 2000; Mattingly & Fleming, 1994). They adjust approaches and use treatment activities that are highly individualized and personalized to the client's particular situation and needs (Guidetti & Tham, 2002; Mattingly & Fleming, 1994). Occupational therapists convey a belief in the individual client's potential for change and growth (Devereaux, 1984; Gahnstrom-Strandqvist et al., 2000) and structure opportunities for success (Mattingly & Fleming, 1994). Other strategies include touch, sense of humor, and sharing

Table 4-4   Strategies Used by Occupational Therapists to Build Rapport

- Provide clients with choices
- Include client in joint problem solving
- Individualize activities and approaches to client's needs
- Convey belief in client's potential
- Structure opportunities for success
- Joke/use humor
- Share personal stories judiciously (without shifting focus from the client's concerns)
- Touch therapeutically

From Cole and McLean (2003), Devereaux (1984), Gahnstrom-Strandqvist et al. (2000), Guidetti & Tham (2002), Mattingly & Fleming (1994), and Taylor (2008).

personal stories to create bonds (Devereaux, 1984; Mattingly & Fleming, 1994; Taylor, 2008).

Strategies may vary by setting. For example, occupational therapists rated rapport and counseling skills significantly higher in developing a therapeutic relationship in adult practice areas than in pediatric settings (Cole & McLean, 2003). In contrast, pediatric and geriatric occupational therapists rated therapeutic touch significantly higher for developing a therapeutic relationship.

Demonstrating Empathy and Rapport in Play

With a foundational understanding of the child, the occupational therapist is able to demonstrate empathy and rapport therapeutically by playing *with* the child (Blanche, 2008; Price & Miner, 2007; Spitzer, 2008). Most pediatric clients cannot conceptually understand a verbal or nonverbal acknowledgment of empathy, and thus, empathy must be demonstrated. Through the therapist's actions, the child can experience empathy and develop feelings of rapport. Engaging in play with the child demonstrates the therapist's understanding of the experience of play. As an adult, the occupational therapist may demonstrate playfulness by being gregarious, uninhibited, comedic, dynamic, creative, and spontaneous (Barnett, 2007; Guitard, Ferland, & Dutil, 2005). By taking on the role of player, the occupational therapist demonstrates an authentic understanding of the joy of play (Bracegirdle, 1992). The occupational therapist can share in play by taking a full role as a player—taking turns, being a character, and being a playmate who assists, supports, and encourages the child, and expresses/mirrors

the child's reactions in ways that promote play. The occupational therapist can enlist family members to assist with playful activities. By playing, the occupational therapist creates a playful environment where pediatric clients can play (Ferland, 2005). This social aspect of play promotes a therapeutic relationship between the occupational therapist and pediatric client, who are engaged together in the activity at hand. The occupational therapist shares in the control, spontaneity, challenge, and possibility of play.

Sharing Control. In assuming a playmate role, the occupational therapist builds rapport by sharing control with the pediatric client and family. The occupational therapist minimizes directiveness to the extent possible for each individual child. An occupational therapist can also share control through flexibly offering choices (what, when, how) and encouraging and accepting the child's reactions to and feelings expressed about the activities (Fleming, 1994; Mattingly & Fleming, 1994; Parham, 1992; Price & Miner, 2007; Yerxa, 1967). For example, a child who is feeling fatigued or taxed during a session may lie down and pretend to be "asleep." Sometimes giving those children the break they need by allowing them to "sleep" or by "sleeping" next to them for a few seconds until the "alarm" goes off is just what they need. In this way, the occupational therapist shares a playful rest moment rather than allowing avoidance or directing the child back to work.

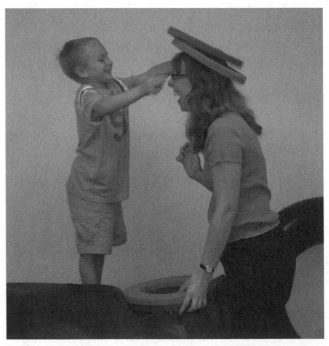

When playing *with* the child, the occupational therapist is a full partner in the activity.

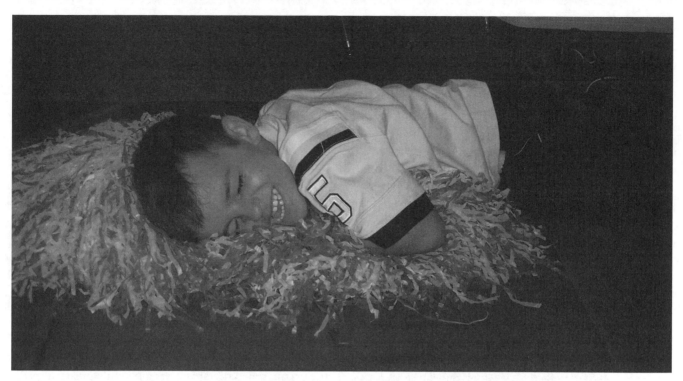

When a child pretends to be asleep, the occupational therapist can become very directive and urge him "back to _____," or he or she may opt to playfully allow a brief pretend sleep break and then use a pretend alarm to wake him up.

The occupational therapist can also share control with family members or other caregivers who may contribute some wonderful ideas for play with this child. When the occupational therapist shares control with clients, clients can also have some sense of internal control and experience the freedom to participate in the spontaneous process of play (Henricks, 1999).

Spontaneity and Flexibility. Although the occupational therapist has a treatment plan and enters each treatment session with plans guided by goals, he or she must remain very flexible in how these plans may be adjusted in the moment of therapy. The occupational therapist must be willing to adjust a treatment plan in the moment to allow spontaneous play opportunities to emerge (Blanche, 2008). Because play is a spontaneous process, and in therapy, a social process as well, the occupational therapist must be open to adapting to the child's response and to seizing upon playful opportunities. The occupational therapist must have a "playful eye" to recognize playful possibilities, such as the example with Michael illustrates.

Managing Challenge. The playful occupational therapist demonstrates empathy for the challenges as well as the joys of play. The occupational therapist can model playful

acceptance of mistakes, errors, trips, falls, and so on. In these circumstances, an adult has a tendency to simply clean up, pick up, fix the mistake, or try again in a quick manner and continue on with the activity at hand. This often happens so swiftly that the child fails to notice it. By slowing down and explicating the process, the occupational therapist can use this as an opportunity to model a sharing of frustration: "Oops, I dropped it" and an "Oh well, that's okay, let's keep playing" attitude. The occupational therapist deliberately reacts in words and actions to demonstrate empathy with the child. The degree of these actions must be graded and matched with the child's developmental level so as not to be interpreted as belittling. The objective is to persist with the playful process rather than become overly preoccupied with the observable product or performance, an extrinsic standard.

Focusing on Future Possibilities. The playful occupational therapist also builds rapport with a child by focusing on the transformative possibility of play. The therapist acts "as if" the pediatric client is not disabled, especially not in the social sense in which disability is understood. The playful occupational therapist is not limited by the realities of current time and space, but feels free to act as if things were different. Thus, the occupational therapist maintains

Michael and Playful Therapeutic Opportunities

Michael was a 4-year-old diagnosed with Pervasive Developmental Disorder. One of his goals for occupational therapy was to write horizontal, vertical, and circular lines. When he was given a writing utensil, he often threw it; at most, he would scribble briefly. Michael threw tantrums when adults would direct control of the writing utensil. He preferred to use nontoy objects and resisted the therapist's suggestions. He seemed most interested in seeing things fall apart or making another big impact—such as throwing, kicking, stepping on, or dumping toys from bins and boxes. His occupational therapist was having difficulty finding a way to work on his prewriting goal and had run out of ideas. During a session, Michael picked up a spray bottle of water and began spraying it repetitively on the table. At first, his occupational therapist thought she should stop this action because it seemed to be very repetitive and to serve no therapeutic purpose. But she carefully ran through his goals in her head for possible ways of intersecting therapeutic goals and this sudden interest. She quickly realized they could use a pencil on the laminated table and then wipe it up with the water. She dried the table off with a quick sweep and managed to get Michael to wait momentarily while she quickly drew a line on the table. "Zip!" she said. Then she pointed to the table and said, "Spray it." He did, and she wiped off the water with a towel. "It's gone! Magic," she said. "Yeah!" he said. Then she offered him a pencil, demonstrating and encouraging him to make different lines, which he did, "erasing" them with water between trials with great exclamations of enjoyment. He kept indicating a desire to continue practicing in this manner. Michael's occupational therapist found herself surprised by the direction the session had gone because she had never anticipated such a therapeutic treatment activity. She also felt a great sense of satisfaction and confidence in her abilities. It was moments like these that affirmed her skill in and belief in the profession. She had identified a way for Michael to learn a skill that he needed in a way that affirmed his interests. This was the first time he drew lines; later, he began practicing on fogged-up windows of the car and other surfaces, and eventually paper.

Learning Activity

Consider the case of Michael:

- Would you feel comfortable using the same occupational therapy approach?
- How else could the occupational therapist have demonstrated empathy and rapport in addressing the client's needs playfully?

is usually the receiver of help for most activities helps the therapist with creative ideas for decorating a new tray table. A child with autism who rarely initiates ideas or social interaction or engages in pretend play suddenly repetitively says "Power Rangers," her brothers' favorite television show, and the occupational therapist then acts as if the child is a Power Ranger. A child who frequently hurts other children and breaks toys because of her poor body awareness and difficulty grading force becomes a super hero who saves people from the "bad guys." When the occupational therapist uses a playful approach, pediatric clients can imagine and explore a different occupational identity of "what if I were _____, what if I could do _____."

Reflective Self-Awareness: Knowing and Managing Playmate and Therapist Roles

A prerequisite for therapeutic use of self is the occupational therapist's self-awareness of attitudes, abilities, limitations, and needs. Occupational therapists must know what their abilities are in order to have and demonstrate confidence in their abilities (Frank, 1958; Lloyd & Maas, 1991). Likewise, occupational therapists must be aware of their limitations to experience and demonstrate humility about their limitations and their relative role in the therapeutic process (Frank, 1958; Mosey, 1986). They must have knowledge of their own needs to address and meet these needs outside of therapy sessions so they do not interfere with focusing on the client's needs within therapy (Lloyd & Maas, 1991; Mosey, 1986; Taylor, 2008). An occupational therapist must be aware of his or her own attitudes and biases to keep them in check when working with clients (Lloyd & Maas, 1991; Punwar, 2000; Taylor, 2008). By being aware of who he or she is, the occupational therapist can control his or her impulses and behaviors to approach clients in a consciously therapeutic manner. The reader is referred to Taylor's work (2008) for detailed guidance on developing self-awareness for promoting therapeutic use of self.

a future orientation (Price & Miner, 2007; Schafer, 1994). This happens most frequently when a child with a significant disability is enabled to take on an extraordinary role. For example, a child with spastic cerebral palsy who

For the play that occurs in a session to be therapeutic, occupational therapists must also know themselves and control their own responses within the session (Schwartzberg, 1993). The therapist must stay focused on the child, determine what response is therapeutic for the child in that moment, and respond accordingly. Responses based on the therapists' own needs and interests may not be therapeutic for the child. When integrating playmate and therapist roles in pediatrics, occupational therapists frequently are faced with their own attitudes about various types of play and the constraints of the physical and social context within which therapy is conducted. With conscious attention to these factors, an occupational therapist can develop his or her individual play style.

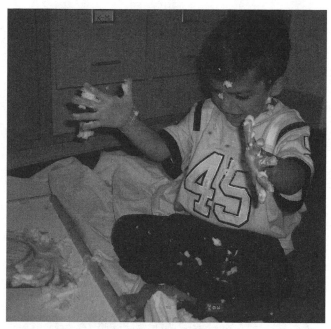

With messy play, occupational therapists must be prepared for the physical impact of the mess as well as be able to suspend rules about neatness and any negative attitudes about messiness.

Learning Activity

Use the worksheet in **Appendix 4-2** to assist you in developing insight and awareness regarding your own values and predispositions related to play.

Managing Therapist Attitudes and Beliefs About Play

Shaped by their personal experiences and values, occupational therapists have their own attitudes about different types of play—about what is and what is not appropriate and about what children should and should not do. It is important that occupational therapists recognize these attitudes as their own so they can focus on being therapeutic when such types of play emerge in therapy sessions. For example, Jacob's occupational therapist did not believe that it was generally appropriate for children to play with "poop," and Michael's occupational therapist did not believe it was generally appropriate for children to write on tables (see above), but both were willing to accept these unconventional actions for their individual therapeutic value in the context of play. Attitudes about power and willingness to share power with clients must be examined to develop a genuine partnership with clients (Palmadottir, 2006), including the child, parents, teachers, and other caregivers. Biases about the child's behavior, parenting approaches, culture, and teaching style must be controlled so that clients can be approached in a nonjudgmental manner (Punwar, 2000).

Attitudes About Humor in Play. Because humor is relative, many people have different attitudes about what constitutes humor. For example, using a made-up robotic

"accent" may be funny, but using an accent typical for a particular social class, geographical region, or ethnic group may be seen as objectionable. A child may focus purely on the difference in sound and be unaware of social attitudes or political backgrounds. Or, the child may be attempting to make sense of social differences. Occupational therapists must be able to set aside their own attitudes to judge objectively the child's intent and others' reception of potentially humorous actions.

Attitudes About Gendered Play. Gendered play is another form of play about which various attitudes abound. As described in Chapter One, research indicates that boys and girls tend to play in segregated groups, playing different activities; however, this is not absolute and may vary to greater and lesser degrees in local sociocultural contexts (Jarrett, Farokhi, Young, & Davies, 2001; Thorne, 1993; Tietz & Shine, 2001; Van Rheenen, 2001). Furthermore, gender boundaries are often negotiated in play (Thorne, 1993; Van Rheenen, 2001). Some people feel most comfortable when children play in traditional gender-based activities, but some find it objectionable. Some people feel comfortable with and even prefer to see girls playing with stereotypically masculine toys, games, and physical activities, but some people object to girls doing some or all aspects of "boy play." Some people enjoy seeing boys play with stereotypically feminine toys, games, and activities (such as dolls, dance, and jump rope), and some are troubled by this. Some people's attitudes vary based on

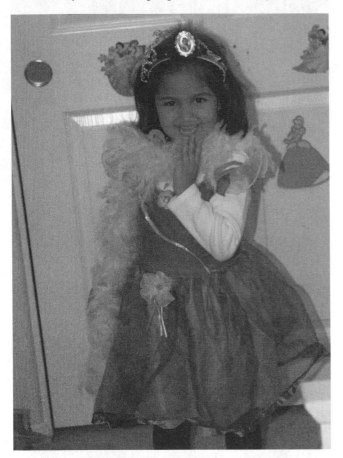

the particular activity or the child's disability. Some worry about a child with a disability being limited or stigmatized by engaging in gendered or cross-gendered play. People may have such attitudes based on their experiences, values, or concerns about society's reactions. Occupational therapists need to recognize that gendered play does exist but is also negotiated in the local social context in the family and on the playground. We have a responsibility to analyze our own attitudes and recognize how they may differ from the available knowledge base (see Chapter One). This enables us to focus on the child, the family, and the social context in an informed manner when analyzing the therapeutic benefits and challenges of gendered or cross-gendered play for an individual client.

Attitudes About Aggressive-Themed Play. Aggressive-themed play is another type of play that commonly evokes strong attitudes. Although many adults are quick to condemn aggression in any form, it is important to note that aggressive behavior and themes are common in typically developing children's play. As described in Chapter One, there are patterns of aggressive-themed play. Researchers have suggested a variety of potential beneficial functions of aggressive play, but there is no agreement about whether aggressive play should be allowed or discouraged. Adults tend to have negative attitudes about aggressive play and at best tolerate it but rarely encourage it (Goldstein, 1995; Johnson, Welteroth, & Corl, 2001). Adult attitudes tend to be related to their educational status, their play memories,

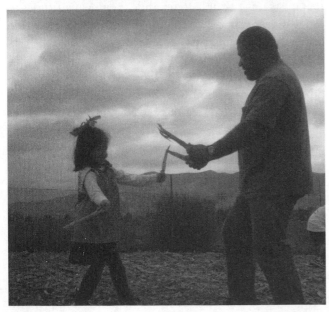

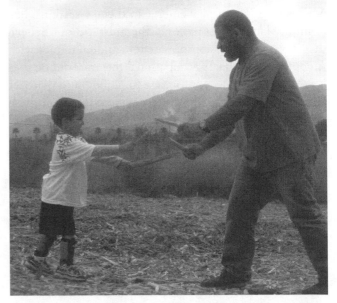

Occupational therapists must examine their own attitudes regarding gendered, cross-gendered, and aggressive-themed play, which commonly occur in children.

presence of siblings, and the child's gender (Goldstein, 1995; Johnson et al., 2001). Recognizing the difference between our attitudes and the knowledge base allows us to focus on individual cases of aggressive play and whether to allow, encourage, discourage, or shape its form.

Managing Physical and Social Constraints

When acting as a child's playmate in an occupational therapy session, the therapist must be aware of physical and social constraints. For example, a child may want to engage in physical play with the therapist, but the therapist must be mindful of his or her own body mechanics to ensure personal safety. Some children want to take risks without recognizing the almost certain danger involved. Another child may find it a game to make large chalk drawings all over the sidewalk, but the school administration may only have designated a particular area for this purpose. The child may find it fun to smear paint all over her body, getting it on her clothes and surrounding furniture, but a parent or program administrator may not be amused given the temporary, if not permanent, damage to physical property. The child may be drawn to loud noises and a loud, excited voice from the therapist, but this may be disruptive to others. In these and similar cases, the occupational therapist might have to leave the playmate role and redirect and set limits for the child to protect self, client, property, or professional relationships in order to safeguard the future of therapy sessions.

Learning to Play in Therapy

Play is about having fun, a pleasurable emotional state (Apter, 1991; Guitard et al., 2005; Holmes, 1999; Skard & Bundy, 2008; see also Chapters One and Two). It is difficult for the child to have fun if the occupational therapist is not having fun. The occupational therapist can play within the therapy session by adopting key features of playfulness: intrinsic motivation, internal control, and freedom to suspend reality (Skard & Bundy, 2008).

Intrinsic Motivation. To tap into their own intrinsic motivation, occupational therapists must identify what they themselves enjoy about being a practitioner and what they like about their individual clients. To be playful, it is especially important to identify the fun aspects. Then, occupational therapists can keep these ideas foremost in their thinking to promote a playful disposition, a real enjoyment of their chosen profession. Therapy can also be very demanding and challenging at times, which can make it difficult to stay intrinsically motivated. Specifically identifying the fun characteristics and reminding oneself of these can help the occupational therapist maintain a genuine playful orientation and a desire or want to be engaged in the session.

Internal Control. Internal control is not to be confused with having total control of the session, because control must be shared with the client as well. Internal control is having confidence in the therapeutic process and one's self as a therapeutic agent, which allows the occupational therapist comfort with sharing control with the child. Each occupational therapist must examine his or her abilities and doubts to identify a plan to build a sense of internal control. With a foundation of theory, research, training, and mentoring, you will know what to do, when to do it, and why you do what you do. Although the details may be specifically enacted with individual clients, the guiding principles and techniques remain stable. You will have the ability to make well-reasoned clinical decisions and determine when modifications to a standard practice are needed. With skill in activity analysis, the cornerstone of therapy, you will have the internal control you need in order to be spontaneous and playful as you share control with your pediatric clients.

Suspending Reality. Occupational therapists who adopt a playful style temporarily suspend their own reality. Play creates a protective frame (Apter, 1991). They are free to be spontaneous and creative (Guitard et al., 2005). They act "as if" free from their own worries, from social conventions, from the apparent limits of clinical "disability," and from planned activities (Spitzer, 2008). The focus is on the child's capacity to do despite disability (Hasselkus & Dickie, 1994; Yerxa, 1967). Play is a transformative process where players transform themselves and their environments, either physically or symbolically, creating meaning for their lives (Henricks, 1999).

As seen in the example of Michael and writing on the table, the playful occupational therapist also acts as if free from social conventions—conventional ideas about both play for the child and appropriate adult-therapist behavior. Michael's occupational therapist was able to suspend social rules about "not writing on the table," enabling him to develop the skills to write; she opted to work on conventional rules later. Conventional ideas often involve demonstrating good disciplined behavior, which is polite and respectful to adults. But if the occupational therapist is going to play with the child, then some of these social rules may have to be held in abeyance. Crawling around on the floor, making exaggerated facial expressions, talking in a sing-song fashion, taking turns in a game, getting dressed up, and many other strategies are not generally accepted as mature professional behavior, and the occupational therapist cannot be overly preoccupied with these social normative ideas during sessions. The playful occupational therapist is free to be silly and laugh without worrying about looking silly even in front of parents, student interns, or other professionals. Instead, the playful occupational therapist recognizes that using these strategies in the context of a playful session is masterful.

The occupational therapist must also distance him- or herself from the realities of life outside the session. The occupational therapist cannot allow him- or herself to be preoccupied with personal finances, an upcoming vacation, family relationships, his or her own health, chores, work relationships, productivity demands, and so forth. All these distractions need to stay outside the session because they take away from the here-and-now quality of the play process.

When occupational therapists play on the boundary of reality and possibility, they take calculated risks. Schafer (1994) argued that this can be very therapeutic because of the potential for reality to be transformed by possibility. However, there is a risk that the potential for growth and development will not materialize. Furthermore, there is always a risk that things might even go "wrong." What might happen if the child gets too disappointed, too frustrated, too disorganized, too angry, or too active? Based on this consideration, the occupational therapist may decide to modify the activity somewhat. This is a balancing act because activities that are too predictable or too safe are unlikely to be very playful or therapeutic. Consider the example of Sarah.

The occupational therapist must calculate the risk that both therapist and client can manage. The occupational therapist is able to abandon neither the reality of the child's life nor the reality of professional responsibility. In other words, the occupational therapist must also remain a therapist and balance therapist and playmate roles.

Developing Your Playful Therapeutic Use of Self: An Ongoing, Reflective Process

Although the development of therapeutic use of self begins with the formal educational training of occupational therapists, it is a lifelong, reflective, demanding, and yet satisfying process. Therapeutic use of self is developed

---

Sarah and a Calculated Risk

Sarah was a 4-year-old client with a seizure disorder and developmental delays who resisted wet, sticky textures in food and in art and learning projects. The occupational therapist suggested she and Sarah play with toy animals, which Sarah liked, in the "mud" (a bowl of chocolate pudding). Sarah appeared excited, repeating the phrase "play with the animals in the mud" until she saw the pudding. She pulled away and directed the therapist, "you do it." The occupational therapist carefully dipped the just-washed animals in the pudding, modeling positive emotions and statements. Soon Sarah came closer and gradually began playing too. At first, she was very careful not to actually touch the pudding, but then it kept happening accidentally. She asked to wipe it off, and the therapist helped her so that she would continue playing. After a few times of wiping the pudding off, the occupational therapist suggested, "you can lick it," and pretended to lick her fingers. Sarah laughed and tried licking the pudding off an animal, deliberately dunking and licking each animal like a spoon. They both laughed. When the occupational therapist described the session to Sarah's mom, Sarah's mom responded, "Yuck!" (pause) "Cool!" This was the first time Sarah had eaten pudding. From then on, Sarah willingly ate pudding with a spoon.

Sarah's occupational therapist planned for this session by washing the animals, anticipating that maybe Sarah might be coaxed into sticking her finger in the pudding and then licking her finger. However, it was in the therapeutic moment that the occupational therapist envisioned a slight modification and allowed Sarah's own unconventional activity modification. The occupational therapist took a calculated risk. She knew the toys were clean and thus safe. She knew this was of great interest to Sarah. She knew this could help promote Sarah's tolerance of tactile sensation. She also knew that many people would frown on a child Sarah's age licking toys that are not meant for licking, especially when she was too old to be mouthing toys (her mother's initial "yuck" response). Her colleagues might even believe it inappropriate, but Sarah's mom was pretty open-minded, frequently commenting that she was willing to try anything that might help Sarah. Sarah's occupational therapist had a playful eye to see this as a therapeutic opportunity. She acted as if free from social rules that might have stopped this activity and its positive therapeutic outcome. This activity also worked because Sarah's occupational therapist considered the fit within Sarah's family context. The therapist was able to recognize the difference between her general social attitudes and the family's and consciously act in a way that was therapeutic. The outcome would not have been so therapeutic if Sarah's family had strict rules about not putting toys in one's mouth, especially if Sarah wanted to play again.

Learning Activity

Consider the case of Sarah:

- Would you be comfortable taking these calculated risks to address therapeutic goals playfully? Why?

- If her family had strict cultural rules about not putting toys in one's mouth, how would you change the treatment activity to address Sarah's needs?

---

throughout our careers through mentoring and reflective practice (Mosey, 1986; Parham, 1987; Price, 2009; Schwartzberg, 1993; Taylor, 2008). This process is highly individualized and personal for each occupational therapist, who must find and develop his or her own therapeutic style. Even with several decades of experience between us, we constantly reflect on practice and find ways to improve each session. Although this process is work, the benefits of a satisfying career are well worth the effort. This is the way occupational therapists elevate practice to an art (Hinojosa, 2007; Mosey, 1981). "Without art, the occupational therapy process is only the application of scientific knowledge in a sterile vacuum" (Mosey, 1981, p. 25).

The need for occupational therapists to develop therapeutic use of self was supported by a study published just as this book was going to press. Taylor et al. (2009) surveyed a random nationwide sample of occupational therapists. Questionnaires were completed by 568 practicing occupational therapists. Although 82–96% valued different aspects of therapeutic use of self, only half felt they were sufficiently trained upon graduation, and less than one-third felt there was sufficient knowledge about therapeutic use of self in occupational therapy. It is our intent and hope that this chapter positively contributes toward this need for professional knowledge and training in pediatric occupational therapy.

To apply the principles and concepts from this book into your practice, you need to integrate these tools with your personal abilities. Throughout this book and accompanying videos are multiple examples of various styles of playful therapeutic interaction.[4] These examples are designed to help you envision what it can be to use oneself as a therapeutic tool. In this particular chapter, a number of specific strategies are presented for building a playful

therapeutic relationship with a pediatric client. The next steps of incorporating these strategies in practice and building your own skills are up to you. It is the reader's responsibility to determine which elements in these examples meet their clients' needs and mesh with their own personhood. "An individual therapeutic style is developed through trying out a variety of different modes of interactions with clients: keeping those that feel right and seem to work, discarding those which do not, and never being afraid to try out a new mode of behavior" (Mosey, 1986, p. 209). Further reflective discussion and observation with experienced and skilled occupational therapists can also yield insight in developing your own therapeutic use of self.

Learning Activity

View the video clips of occupational therapy sessions. As you view these videos, complete the Video Review Form in **Appendix 4-3** to help you increase your understanding of therapeutic use of self in pediatric occupational therapy.

Although some of us may have personal traits that are naturally more or less helpful in healing, our therapeutic use of self is a conscious role that we create and play (Frank, 1958; Taylor, 2008). This therapeutic role can be influenced by, but is not dependent on, who we are (Frank, 1958). Therapeutic use of self is a product of knowledge and skill (Taylor, 2008). Each therapist may have a preferred style that is consistent with our personalities; however, it is important that we become comfortable and able to adjust therapeutic modes for different clients and different situations (Mosey, 1986; Taylor, 2008). For some of us, these play strategies feel very comfortable and natural with children. For others, with a different predisposition, such strategies may be more challenging to assume. Even caring is a skill to be developed (Gilfoyle, 1980). You may need to learn or relearn to play as an adult. You must learn to play with a range of children. Bracegirdle (1992) suggested interacting with playful children, who will teach you to play if you are open to their directions and enticements, and watching playful parents play with their young children, especially babies. By paying conscious attention to developing your skills, trying them, and reflecting on their outcome, you will develop an understanding of the nuances of matching strategies to clients and will hone your skills. With ongoing practice and

---

[4]The video clips and case studies provide a sample of some ways in which play may be included in occupational therapy. Application to other settings and clients is at the discretion of the treating occupational therapist.

analytical reflection, occupational therapists can develop these skills regardless of their individual comfort level and innate disposition.

Therapeutic use of self also involves emotional work. Occupational therapists care for people who are dealing with difficult challenges, traumatic events, and crises (Taylor, 2008). Confronted with repeated exposure to the challenges of life, illness, disability, and sometimes death, occupational therapists often struggle alongside clients and families to make sense of negative events, pain, and suffering (McColl, 2003). Occupational therapists work with people who may be experiencing very difficult emotions such as anxiety, anger, and depression or who may have other challenging interpersonal characteristics (Frank, 1958; Taylor, 2008; Taylor et al., 2009). Sometimes it is hard to understand or face these emotions and behaviors, especially when they can seem like personal attacks. It takes effort to manage our own feelings, responses, and behaviors to focus on the client's therapeutic needs and goals. On top of this, the occupational therapist must constantly attend to and adjust his or her style and responses to each child, and the child's developmental level and unique characteristics. Additionally, occupational therapists may not always get clear positive feedback for their actions because children with disabilities cannot always provide this (Brazelton & Tronick, 1980; Greenspan, & Wieder, 1997). Without this external reinforcing feedback, occupational therapists' efforts can feel more like work and cause us to doubt our efficacy or to become discouraged with our attempts. Sustaining a playful style despite these challenges definitely involves a strong therapeutic use of self for the pediatric occupational therapist.

This intense work is clearly very important and necessary for effective therapy, but it can also cause burnout if occupational therapists do not find ways to care for themselves outside of work (Taylor & Peloquin, 2008). Burnout in occupational therapists has been associated with emotional exhaustion (Schlenz, Guthrie, & Dudgeon, 1995) and the complexity of client problems (Kraeger & Walker, 1993). Therapist strategies of caring for themselves are very individual but may include exercise, talking to a friend or family member, reading fiction, or cooking a favorite meal (Taylor, 2008). For some occupational therapists, counseling or psychotherapy may be helpful to manage feelings ignited in the course of being a therapist. Caring for themselves helps provide occupational therapists with the energy and positive self-concept to care for their clients (Devereax, 1984).

> ### Learning Activity
>
> Reflect on what you need to care for yourself in order to be therapeutic:
> - What helps you to restore your energy?
> - What do you need to do to maintain your physical health and well-being?
> - What do you need to do to promote your mental health and well-being?

The benefits of the work of therapeutic use of self are tremendous in terms of satisfying practice. Occupational therapists report that a harmonious therapeutic relationship with clients is a core aspect of their practice on a daily basis and a source of satisfaction (Hasselkus & Dickie, 1994). Occupational therapists feel competent when working together with clients as partners focused on personally meaningful goals (Gahnstrom-Strandqvist et al., 2000; Rosa & Hasselkus, 1996). The absence of a therapeutic relationship is considered a barrier to practice, which occupational therapists strive to overcome (Hasselkus & Dickie, 1994). Occupational therapists believe that the therapeutic relationship, empathy, and rapport help bring about functional outcomes across practice settings (Cole & McLean, 2003; Taylor et al., 2009). Once an occupational therapist is able to behave playfully and creatively, he or she is more likely also to experience play while working as a therapist (Dunkerley, Tickle-Degnen, & Coster, 1997; Ferland, 2005) and increased job enjoyment (Vergeer & MacRae, 1993). Occupational therapists also feel successful when they "find the key" to helping a child (Case-Smith, 1997, p. 140). A playful relationship is often key to helping a child.

THERAPEUTIC USE OF SELF AND CAREGIVER RELATIONSHIPS

Although this book is committed to the use of play with pediatric clients, pediatric practice is incomplete without also applying therapeutic use of self with the child's family and other adult caregivers. Supporting and including families in treatment planning and intervention are best practices in pediatric occupational therapy (Dunn, 2000; Maternal and Child Health Bureau, 2005). Families want to feel that professionals support them, listen, and understand their needs as a family and do not judge them (Petr & Barney, 1993).In practice, the inclusion of families varies. Brown, Humphry, and Taylor (1997) found that occupational therapists use a hierarchical continuum of the following levels of family-therapy involvement, with each level requiring more knowledge and skill: no family involvement, family as informant, family as therapist's assistant, family as co-client, family as consultant, family as team collaborator, and family as director of service. Occupational therapists have an obligation to commit to supporting and including families at the latter, higher levels. This is not an expectation that families must be involved, but rather that families are welcomed and supported to be as involved as they desire and are able.

Families have individual experiences, routines, strengths, needs, and hopes for the future (Adams, Wilgosh, & Sobsey, 1990; Anderson & Hinojosa, 1984; Cook, 1996; Gallimore, Weisner, Kaufman, & Bernheimer, 1989; Maternal and Child Health Bureau, 2005; Primeau, 1998; Schneider & Gearhart, 1988; Wikler, Wasow, & Hatfield, 1983) that shape the social environment for our clients and therapy. Consequently, the occupational therapist will need a good therapeutic relationship with the child's family, teachers, and other caregivers so they too will feel comfortable, trust the therapist, work with the therapist, and be willing to try different activities with their children.

Sometimes a parent's emotions and behaviors can be incompatible with playfulness or may appear to be obstacles in therapy. As parents adjust to the child's disability, they may experience doubts and guilt about their parenting abilities, stress and anxiety about their child's future, and other negative and complex emotions that change with each stage of the child's development (Anderson &

Hinojosa, 1984). Whenever the occupational therapist presents evaluation results or mentions the child's needs, the parent may experience a resurgence in distress or mourning over the child's deficits. As a result of the parents' feelings, they may be overprotective or highly directive with their children. Parents may need to express these feelings. If they trust the occupational therapist, parents may share these feelings with him or her. Some parents may need additional support and can be referred to counseling or parent support groups.

Sometimes a parent's emotions and behaviors trigger attitudes in the occupational therapist, who may overly identify with the child or the caregiver. This is another aspect of pediatric practice that necessitates that the occupational therapist reflect on and consciously check his or her own reactions in order to remain therapeutic. Most parents and other caregivers benefit when the child's occupational therapist provides nurture and support regarding the challenges they are facing; positive feedback about what they are doing well to reinforce their competence and self-esteem; joint problem solving to promote their own experience of mastery; and information as suggestions to be collaboratively evaluated in relation to the parents' occupations (instead of advice giving, where the parents are expected to submit to the therapist's expertise regardless of readiness, values, and ability) (Anderson & Hinojosa, 1984). Furthermore, a playful approach can be extended to caregivers to emphasize the pleasure of sharing play, with its focus on the child's potential instead of his or her difficulties (Ferland, 2005). These specific strategies for caregivers (**Table 4-5**) can help create a therapeutic relationship that promotes the child's participation in play.

Table 4-5   Strategies for Therapeutic Use of Self With Families and Other Caregivers of Pediatric Clients

- Allow parents to express feelings without judgment.
- Reflect on and consciously check own reactions to caregiver emotions and behaviors.
- Provide nurture and support regarding the challenges they are facing.
- Refer to counseling or support groups when caregiver needs go beyond the therapist's abilities to address.
- Give positive feedback about what they are doing well.
- Engage in joint problem solving.
- Present information as suggestions to be evaluated collaboratively (avoid giving advice).
- Incorporate a playful approach.
- Involve in play activities.

Adapted from Anderson and Hinojosa (1984) and Ferland (2005)

A family's or other caregiver's values and behaviors regarding play and occupational therapy can also be influenced by their cultural and socioeconomic background, which may be both similar to and different from the therapist's personal and professional values. Occupational therapy values are based in predominantly Western, Anglo-American, middle- and upper-class values such as autonomy, personal achievement, and goal-directed individual independence (Awaad, 2003). The medical culture, in which occupational therapists practice, values the professional as expert, measurable and clearly defined procedures and outcomes, and fragmented and specialized service—values that tend to conflict with developing family partnerships (Lawlor & Mattingly, 1998). In contrast, some cultures value religion, family honor, or societal welfare over the focus on an individual (Awaad, 2003). Different cultures may also have different valuations of play. For example, in a study of 33 French and 39 European American 20-month-old children and their mothers, Suizzo and Bornstein (2006) found that French children engaged in more exploratory play, whereas U.S. children engaged in more symbolic play, and French mothers less frequently solicited symbolic play than U.S. mothers.

To develop cultural competence in working with families and other caregivers, occupational therapists must build self-awareness of their own personal and professional culture as well as knowledge about others' cultures (Awaad, 2003; Chiang & Carlson, 2003; Munoz, 2007; Wittman & Velde, 2002). This is not to be confused with developing rules or stereotypes about different cultural groups because a focus on the individual's experiences and values is still important (Awaad, 2003; Chiang & Carlson, 2003). The occupational therapist may ask the family about their background and advise them to notify the therapist if there is something about therapy that does not feel right or fit in with their culture (Munoz, 2007). Given that culture cannot be seen or assumed, it is wise to consistently address culture in this direct manner with all

families regardless of whether they seem culturally similar or dissimilar. Cultural competency involves more than recognizing differences; it also involves consciously respecting these differences (Awaad, 2003; Chiang & Carlson, 2003; Munoz, 2007; Wittman & Velde, 2002) as a form of therapeutic use of self. Awaad (2003) notes that if we do a good activity analysis of occupational meaning, cultural meaning will also be revealed.

Points of similarity must also be recognized for effective therapeutic use of self. For example, in her research with African American families who have children with medical illnesses and disabilities, Mattingly (2006) found that themes from children's popular play culture, such as Disney characters, can create a shared point for health care providers to interact with children and their families despite differences in race, culture, and class.

■ CONCLUSION

Therapeutic use of self is a powerful tool in occupational therapy. In pediatrics, a playful therapeutic use of self is especially important and is used in conjunction with activity analysis to promote play. This chapter focused on how a playful therapeutic use of self promotes a productive therapeutic relationship. The therapist is a model of playfulness for the child. This playful approach engages the client and therapist despite the often difficult work of therapy. With a playful therapeutic use of self, both occupational therapist and child can have fun in occupational therapy. This book provides you with core knowledge, considerations, and strategies to get you started and to help you reflect on your developing skills. We hope that you may revisit this material over time to build and revitalize your playful therapeutic use of self. Next, we examine how occupational therapists apply their knowledge of play and their skills in activity analysis and therapeutic use of self to select and design therapeutic play activities.

Appendix 4-1

Occupational Therapist Pediatric Communication Strategies Checklist

Pediatric Communication Strategies Checklist

Child's Name: _____

	Have You Communicated Playfulness Through This Strategy?	Child's Response* (Positive, Neutral, Negative)	Notes/Comments†
Eyes Look at the child Look between the child and a potential toy/play object			
Face Exaggerate and hold positive emotional expressions, especially surprise, smiles, and concern Imitate the child's expression			
Body Turn toward the child Exaggerate and slow body movements such as imitation, head nodding, head wagging, or head cocking Hold out, manipulate, hide, or point to toys/objects			
Touch To get attention To show toy, action			
Voice (Vocalizations) Use playful tone Vary pitch, loudness, rhythm Repeat sounds Imitate sounds and ways sounds are used by child			
Language Imitate child's words Match language to child's development Use language in song, melody, rhythm, or different voice (e.g., accent) Use "kid play" words, phrases, and sounds Use humor, jokes, and mischievous tone Talk as if toys or body parts were alive and thinking			

Notes: These strategies must occur in a close enough space that the child can notice these actions.

*If the child's response is negative (e.g., agitation, destructiveness, withdrawal, pushing away, fussing, crying), it suggests that currently this is not an effective play communication strategy for him or her. If the child's response is positive (e.g., increased self-initiation, eye contact, affect/smiling, attention, orienting, leaning toward, participation, behavior modulation, vocalizations/communication), it suggests that this is an effective play communication strategy that should be continued for him or her. If the child's response is neutral (no observable response), the strategy cannot be discounted because he or she may respond later if the strategy is tried again.

†You may want to note specific details of the strategies and the child's response.

Appendix 4-2

Occupational Therapist Self-Reflection Form: Playful Therapeutic Use of Self

Self-Reflection Form: Playful Therapeutic Use of Self

This form is designed to help occupational therapists be aware of their own attitudes, knowledge, and abilities related to consciously using themselves as a tool to create a playful therapeutic environment for pediatric clients.

As you consider each statement, think about how this impacts your therapeutic use of self:

1. I am creative in these ways: _____

    _____

2. I would like to be more creative in this way: _____

3. I do (not) know how to play by myself and do (not) enjoy it.

4. To me, the most important type of play is _____.

5. I prefer to play _____.

6. My best remembrances of play as a child are _____.

7. My worst remembrances of play as a child are _____.

8. I do (not) know how to play and enjoy playing with typical children who are infants, toddlers, preschoolers, school-age, and adolescents.

9. I do (not) know how to play and enjoy playing with children who have physical disabilities, developmental disabilities, and psychosocial disabilities.

10. I prefer that children play this type(s) of play: _____

11. I prefer that children play in this way: _____

12. I am uncomfortable when children play this type(s) of play: _____

13. I am uncomfortable when children play in this way: _____

14. What I most dislike about children's play is _____.

15. I am (un)comfortable being silly (exaggerating facial expressions, making up voices/songs, etc.).

16. I am (un)comfortable acting like a child.

17. I am (un)comfortable joking.

18. I am (un)comfortable being close to children.

19. I am (un)comfortable sharing power with a child (not having total control).

20. When another adult is watching, I am (un)comfortable being silly, acting like a child, joking, or playing.

21. I have a good understanding of play for these developmental ages: _____

22. I have a good understanding of these types of play: _____
_____

23. I experience positive therapeutic relationships with these pediatric clients:

_____

_____

24. I am (not) able to adjust my play style to these pediatric clients: _____

_____

25. I feel (un)comfortable waiting for a child's response.

26. I do (not) know the top play preferences for all my pediatric clients.

27. I do (not) enjoy being a pediatric occupational therapist.

28. I do (not) know key techniques for addressing my pediatric clients' needs.

29. I am (not) distracted by external thoughts/concerns when providing therapy with a pediatric client.

30. I believe parents and other caregivers should behave with children in this way:

_____

_____

31. I believe parents and other caregivers should not behave with children in this way:

_____

_____

32. To summarize, I believe my three greatest strengths for playful therapeutic use of self are _____, _____, and _____. The three areas I most need to develop for a playful therapeutic use of self are _____, _____, and _____.

Appendix 4-3

Therapeutic Use of Self Video Review Form for Occupational Therapy Sessions

Therapeutic Use of Self Video Review Form

Directions: Use this form to guide your viewing of the DVD treatment sessions to increase your understanding of therapeutic use of self in pediatric occupational therapy. Complete this form for each treatment session.

How does the therapist communicate playfulness?

Nonverbal strategies:

Verbal strategies:

How did the therapist get and respond to input from the child?

How does the therapist demonstrate empathy and develop rapport with the child?

Were there any physical or social constraints or special challenges with which the therapist had to contend (e.g., attention, opposition, safety, misunderstanding)?

If yes, how were they dealt with?

What aspect of this session did you find most fun?

What aspect of this session would be most challenging for you if you were the therapist?

What might you have done differently?

How was this occupational therapy session similar to and different from the other sessions?

Section Three
...And How to Apply Them

5

Selecting Play Activities: Activity Analysis, Clinical Reasoning, and Frames of Reference

After reading this chapter the reader will

1. Identify the processes of clinical reasoning.

2. Identify common pediatric frames of reference.

3. Describe how activity analysis, clinical reasoning, and frames of reference impact activity selection.

4. Select appropriate activities based on clinical reasoning using frames of reference and activity analysis.

Children at play are not playing about. Their games should be seen as their most serious minded activity.
—Michel de Montaigne

In Chapter Three, we highlighted the importance of activity analysis as a primary tool of occupational therapy. In this chapter, we will demonstrate how activity analysis, clinical reasoning, and the specific lens of a chosen frame of reference intersect and allow us to select playful activities that are "just right." We examine the clinical reasoning process used by occupational therapists and provide an overview of the commonly used frames of reference as a backbone for our discussion of the use of selection strategies within treatment sessions.

The process of activity selection considers both frames of reference and clinical reasoning. Clinical reasoning allows therapists to select the appropriate frame of reference that in turns guides our activity analysis and activity selection. Knowledge of the specific features of activities gained through general activity analysis helps therapists to choose treatment activities well matched to the client's needs and desires. Clinical reasoning always plays an important role

in guiding intervention choices. The interaction between the different forms of clinical reasoning enables us to consider varied aspects of a client's needs all at once and to evaluate the possibilities for intervention and their potential benefits. Thus, before we can discuss the process of activity selection, we must begin with an overview of clinical reasoning followed by a discussion of the various frames of reference relevant to pediatric practice.

■ CLINICAL REASONING

What is clinical reasoning? Of the many definitions of clinical reasoning, we use the one proposed by Schell (2003): Clinical reasoning is the "process used by practitioners to plan, direct, perform, and reflect on client care" (Schell, 2003, p. 131). Why is it important? Until recently, therapists were unable to explain how and why they made the decisions they made in practice. How can occupational therapists improve practice and teach practice to students and novice therapists if we cannot clearly delineate our decision-making processes during therapeutic interventions? We should be able to clearly articulate why we choose what we choose to do in therapy. Prior to the early 1980s, it was identified that a better understanding of the reasoning process was clearly needed (Schell & Schell, 2008). A Slagle lecture by Joan Rogers in the early 1980s brought this problem to the attention of the community of occupational therapists. Then, in a collaborative effort between the American Occupational Therapy Association and the American Occupational Therapy Foundation, two researchers, Mattingly and Fleming, working with an expert in reflective practice, initiated a study of the decision-making processes of therapists (Schell & Schell, 2008). What they found, which has been confirmed in multiple studies since, is that therapists do not use one process of reasoning; they use many (Mattingly & Fleming, 1994).

The aspects of clinical reasoning identified in the occupational therapy literature include scientific, pragmatic, procedural, interactive, narrative, ethical, and conditional reasoning (Case-Smith, Richardson, & Schultz-Krohn, 2005; Mattingly & Fleming, 1994; Schell, 2003; Schell & Schell, 2008). Typically in practice, occupational therapists engage in multiple forms of reasoning at once as they decide on a course of action. Occupational behavior is complex, and our problem solving and decision making for any particular client or situation require flexible thinking and consideration of a wide range of factors that may influence any situation. The different forms of clinical reasoning individually are more or less appropriate for specific issues and circumstances. In varied combinations, they guide us to make decisions in any practice situation.

Occupational therapists engage in scientific clinical reasoning when making decisions based on evidence, clinical knowledge, and experience. Scientific reasoning uses logical methods, including theory-based decision making, hypothesis testing, and statistical evidence (Schell & Schell, 2008). You can see your own scientific reasoning at work when you consider the diagnosis of the client you are working with and consider both what theory would suggest and what typically happens when you work with a client such as this one. You use scientific reasoning when you utilize the play research presented earlier in this book to make decisions in therapy. Some authors consider diagnostic reasoning a subcategory of scientific clinical reasoning (Schell & Schell, 2008).

Pragmatic reasoning takes into consideration the practical reality of the situation. Occupational therapists consider the materials, resources, and environmental supports available to them as they make decisions (Case-Smith et al., 2005). Occupational therapists also consider their own personal situation and skill. Pragmatic reasoning enters into decisions as we consider all the factors not specific to the client but to the situation. Pragmatic reasoning is used in situations where the practice setting may determine certain priorities for intervention; for example, in a school setting, educational activities take precedent. You may note this form of reasoning yourself when you decide to use one intervention approach over another because of the equipment you have or do not have available to you, or to use the new knowledge you have based on a course you just attended. You may also see yourself thinking pragmatically when you

consider your service delivery options and client scheduling within the reality of your caseload and workday.

Procedural reasoning is typically used when occupational therapists choose specific therapeutic intervention routines for a specific condition. This form of reasoning may or may not be based in science or evidence. It may be merely habit or "what is done" at a particular facility. This form of reasoning often is driven by diagnosis. You may see yourself using this form of reasoning if you choose a specific form of intervention with a child based on his or her diagnosis because you believe this intervention is effective for a particular diagnostically driven symptom.

Interactive reasoning is the thinking that permits collaboration with a client and fosters therapeutic relationships. In the interactive reasoning process, occupational therapists seek to know and understand the interests of the child and what she or he perceives as fun and meaningful. Interactive reasoning is the key to discovering who the clients are and what they find motivating. As such, interactive reasoning relies heavily on therapeutic use of self (see Chapter Four). You will note your own use of interactive reasoning when you are empathetic with your client, concern yourself with his or her likes and dislikes, and use all of your verbal and nonverbal behaviors to collaborate with your client and encourage his or her participation (Case-Smith et al., 2005; Schell & Schell, 2008).

Narrative reasoning enables occupational therapists to consider the child within all of his or her varied roles and across the contexts of home, school, and community. This type of reasoning is used in understanding the occupational profile of the child (Schell, 2003; Schell & Schell, 2008). The narrative process enables the therapist to understand where the child came from, his or her history, and as his or her present level of function and future goals (Bryze, 2008). You may note your own use of this form of reasoning as you consider a client's culture and the influence of this on the current situation, or as you imagine his or her future and try to anticipate how the client's current condition will impact that future.

Ethical reasoning allows occupational therapists to consider an ethical dilemma from many alternative directions (Schell & Schell, 2008). In pediatric practice, it may help therapists weigh the risks and benefits of an intervention or prioritize service allocation (Case-Smith et al., 2005). In combination with scientific reasoning, ethical reasoning allows occupational therapists to weigh evidence of efficacy while also considering the ethical implications of using certain approaches. Ethical reasoning is also used when three therapists call out sick, and not every client can be seen that day. Somehow individuals must be prioritized for service. You will find yourself using this form of reasoning as you try to determine the "right" thing to do in your day-to-day practice.

Finally, conditional reasoning allows more experienced therapists to envision multiple possible outcomes and to look beyond the present activity choice, blending all forms of reasoning (Schell & Schell, 2008). Conditional reasoning enables the therapist to consider past experiences, present information, and the many possible futures to link intervention today with the long-term goal of tomorrow for each individual child.

Occupational therapists flow back and forth between the different forms of clinical reasoning depending on the situation they are in and the types of decision making required at the moment. Therapists use different reasoning when deciding their schedule for the day versus deciding which course to attend to further their knowledge and expand their competence. A different type of reasoning may be used when deciding which evaluation methods to engage in with a child or when trying to choose a specific activity in the moment to engage a child to meet a goal. The remainder of this chapter will consider how clinical reasoning allows occupational therapists to choose the appropriate frame of reference to use at any given time during assessment and intervention for a child.

■ FRAMES OF REFERENCE

Frames of reference are "a set of interrelated internally consistent concepts, definitions and postulates that provide a systematic description of and prescription for a practitioner's interaction within a particular aspect of a profession's domain of concern" (Mosey, 1981, p. 129). Frames of reference are based on theory and relate theory to practice (Dunbar, 2007; Kramer & Hinojosa, 1999). They are organizational structures for theory that provide information for problem identification and intervention options, as well as a common language to guide practice decisions (Dunbar, 2007; Kramer & Hinojosa, 1999).

In pediatric occupational therapy practice, frames of reference are used to guide both evaluation and intervention (Kramer & Hinojosa, 1999; Law, Missiuna, Pollock, & Stewart, 2005). They provide the lens through which the child's functional capacity is viewed. Just as one can put on and take off different glasses depending on the current need, such as using reading and distance glasses at different times, so too can one use multiple frames of reference. Throughout the rest of the chapter, we want you to think of frames of reference as lenses through which you view a child's behavior. These lenses then help in the activity selection process for intervention by providing guidelines for choosing types of activities, equipment, techniques and strategies, environments, and possible outcomes (Law et al., 2005). There are many good resources available that explain frames of reference in depth. This section is meant as a summary overview to remind the reader of each frame's core principles and their relationship to activity analysis and activity selection. With that said, let us examine our choices of which glasses to wear and our reasoning for when to wear them.

> ### Learning Activity
>
> As you read through the section on frames of reference, consider which form(s) of clinical reasoning you might engage in while selecting a particular frame.

Occupation-Based Frames of Reference

Occupation-based frames of reference are based on contemporary systems theory and take an integrated approach to evaluation and intervention (Law et al., 2005). Occupation-based frames of reference are often selected when increased immediate participation in a specific activity is targeted. These approaches incorporate both general and dynamic systems concepts such as interaction and complexity between parts of the system; motivation and meaning; manipulation of constraints; activity engagement in multiple contexts; and repetition and practice (Law et al., 2005). Common approaches used in pediatric therapy include the acquisition, motor learning, and cognitive frames of reference.

The acquisition frame of reference is based on theories of learning and behavior and is commonly used in occupational therapy to address learning-specific skills (Law et al., 2005; Royeen & Duncan, 1999). Intervention therefore includes teaching and learning techniques via direct instruction, engagement, and repetition of an identified activity that is difficult to the child (Law et al., 2005). Motor learning places particular emphasis on motor patterns and synergies used by the child, and facilitation of intrinsic and extrinsic feedback through knowledge of results and performance while practicing the movement goal. Cognitive approaches focus on the development of motor skills through cognitive strategy use in context (Law et al., 2005; Polatajko & Mandich, 2004).

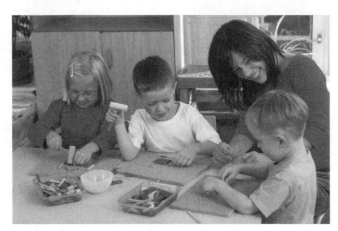

Direct instruction can be used to address specific skills.

Neuromaturation-Based Frames of Reference

Neuromaturation-based frames of reference are chosen when occupational therapists seek to strengthen underlying foundational abilities in a client to allow greater occupational performance to emerge. These frames of reference operate with an underlying assumption that therapeutic activity can change the inherent skills and abilities of the child, and by changing these skills, overall function and engagement in broad areas of occupation also improve (Law et al., 2005). Although these frames of reference were originally derived from a developmental or maturational/stage theory standpoint and a hierarchical view of the nervous system, literature regarding some of these frames of reference has begun to incorporate the newer concepts of neuroscience and a heterarchical view of the nervous system (Bundy & Murray, 2003; Howle, 2002; Spitzer, 1999). Common neuromaturation-based frames of reference used in pediatric occupational therapy practice include neurodevelopmental treatment (NDT) and Ayres' Sensory Integration (ASI) theory and treatment. These frames of reference tend to have very specific guidelines for assessment and intervention, thus requiring specific knowledge and often advanced training to fully understand the use of these approaches.

NDT is a sensorimotor frame of reference that is often used in children with neurological or muscular disorders (Schoen & Anderson, 1999). This approach to intervention is focused on postural control, motor coordination, and careful analysis of the child's movement patterns. Developed by Berta and Karl Bobath in the 1940s, NDT has expanded to include principles of motor learning and dynamic systems perspectives (Howle, 1997, 2002; Law et al., 2005). With the addition of these principles, intervention using an NDT approach not only focuses on motoric

characteristics of the child but also places emphasis on the task, motivation, environment, and function (Howle, 2002). The outcome of an activity according to this frame of reference depends on an interaction between the child, environment, and task (Schoen & Anderson, 1999), but the focus of the intervention is on bringing about change in the child's skill to enhance performance.

The Ayres' Sensory Integration theory and treatment was originally developed in the 1950s by Dr. A. Jean Ayres. Ayres continued to work on and refine the theory, assessment tools including the Southern California Sensory Integration Test (SCIT) and the Sensory Integration and Praxis Test (SIPT), and treatment strategies for children with SI dysfunction until her death in 1988 (Ayres, 2005; Kramer & Hinojosa, 1999; Law et al., 2005). Since 1988, there have been numerous contributions by other occupational therapists to this frame of reference; however, the major concepts related to intervention initially articulated by Ayres have remained.

As a child-directed approach, the Ayres' Sensory Integration treatment creates opportunities for the child to actively participate in play that provides controlled and specific sensory input[1]. The goal of these experiences is an adaptive response that indicates that the child is integrating sensory information. Again, although improved function and participation in occupation is ultimately what is expected as an outcome when using an SI frame of reference, the experiences are typically aimed at addressing the inherent sensory processing abilities within the child.

■ PULLING IT ALL TOGETHER

Within any specific direct therapy session, occupational therapists must choose how to spend time with the child. As we have stated, activity analysis is an important tool in the process of understanding the qualities of any activity. Once skilled at this process, occupational therapists quickly consider each potential activity, determine the features of the activity that may be used therapeutically, and use clinical reasoning to make the decision regarding the appropriateness of the particular activity at that moment, based on the frame of reference selected.

The use of activity analysis, clinical reasoning, and appropriate frames of reference for selection of activities is a circular and ongoing process. Like any dynamic system, therapeutic intervention with another human being is complex, and a change in one part of the system

[1]see *www.siglobalnetwork.org*

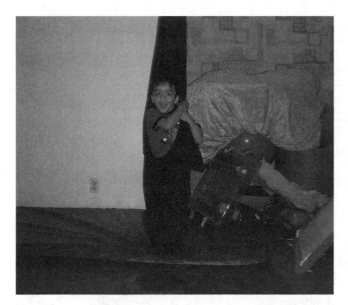 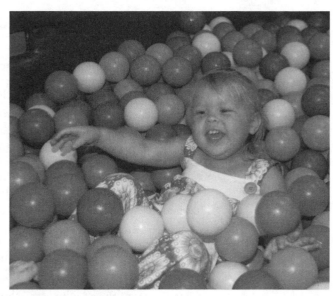

The SI frame of reference uses appropriate sensory inputs to assist a child in making adaptive responses to novel challenges.

(e.g., context) may require change in another part (e.g., service delivery or specific frame of reference). We have tried to pull the process apart and write about it in a linear way to make it more clear and understandable; however, intervention sessions are fluid, and the child's reactions to any of our prior intervention decisions may alter our reasoning and change our next decision in the blink of an eye. Experienced therapists make these intervention decisions quickly, on the spur of the moment, to allow playful interactions to occur in a therapeutic way. The comment, "it looks like you are just playing" is common when observing expert pediatric occupational therapists in their sessions as they rapidly make adjustments and select appropriate activities. However, it should be clear that there is a substantial amount of clinical reasoning going on inside the therapist's head to make it look so easy.

As you may have gathered, there are many things to be considered in making these activity decisions. The different forms of clinical reasoning are important in this process (**Table 5-1**). Because of our focus on play in this book, we highlight again the importance of interactive reasoning in activity selection. If occupational therapists wish to make therapy playful and fun and to focus on play as an important occupation to promote and encourage, they must use interactive reasoning to choose activities that are meaningful to the client.

So how do occupational therapists actually select activities? When first learning, it is often helpful to carefully consider each of the child's goals, select the appropriate frame of reference, and plan a variety of activities to reach those goals. However, as you will discover in pediatric practice, sometimes children have other ideas. All of your plans can quickly go down the drain if a child comes in and has had a rough morning or is not feeling well. Sometimes the child will request a particular activity, and you may want to consider using it in that moment. So you then must either quickly do a general activity analysis of the chosen activity in your head, or use knowledge you have already based on earlier completion of the general activity analysis. As we have stated, the general activity analysis provides an in-depth look at the demands of the activity. Next, using the appropriate forms of clinical reasoning, you must consider what was learned from a general task analysis of the activity demands and match that to what is known about the child's abilities and the occupational therapy goals. Let us consider how this works in the case of Tiffany.

If the occupational therapist selects the particular activity (in Tiffany's case, it would be finger-painting), then she or he will prioritize which aspects of the activity demands will be emphasized to provide the most therapeutic benefit at that moment. The activity begins and is observed. At this point, the process of client-focused activity analysis begins, which is ongoing at every moment when working with a client. The therapist continually observes and adapts, changes the activity in some way, or scraps it and starts another. But with all the things that can be observed, what are we observing for?

General activity analysis does not use a particular frame of reference because it provides a detailed analysis of a specific activity that is unrelated to a particular client. Occupational therapists do use frames of reference when

Table 5-1 Questions and Considerations for Activity Selection Based on Clinical Reasoning

Type of Reasoning	Questions and Considerations During Activity Selection
Scientific	What frames of reference can and should be used to plan intervention activities for this child?
	Does this activity "fit" this particular frame of reference? Does this activity address the problem that I have hypothesized is the issue for this child?
	What is the scientific evidence regarding the effectiveness and safety of the activity?
Pragmatic	What setting am I practicing in? Does that influence my choice of activities in any way? Are there games and activities that cannot be engaged in?
	What materials and resources are available?
	Do I have the proper space to do this activity safely?
Interactive	What is fun and meaningful for the child?
	What does this child like and enjoy?
	In what aspects of the activity is the child most interested?
Narrative	What are the child's roles at home, school, and in the community, and what activities are associated with them?
	What are the goals identified by the child and the family?
Ethical	What are the risks and benefits of the potential therapeutic activity?
	Am I equipped and trained to select, use, and adapt this type of therapeutic activity?
Conditional	What is the possible future for this child, and could the activity choice help the child toward reaching that possible future?
Procedural	What activities are typically selected for individuals with this diagnosis?

Adapted from Schell & Schell, 2008

Tiffany and Finger-Painting

Tiffany is a 3½-year-old girl with a diagnosis of Down syndrome. As the occupational therapist for the school, you are in the classroom frequently. You have made the following observations of Tiffany during your evaluation and subsequent visits to her class.

Tiffany is generally a pleasant girl, but she can be strong willed. She has friends in her classroom, and she enjoys being with and playing with her peers. She typically wants to do the same activities in the classroom that her peers are doing.

She enjoys movement when it does not require extensive endurance. For example, you were told that at home, she loves to swing on the porch swing, but she does not often play chase games with her peers outside, and she avoids the playground swings at school, which require her to sit with minimal support. Similarly, Tiffany has difficulty maintaining an upright seated position for any period of time, often slumping in her chair.

She has difficulty orienting clothing appropriately and often loses her balance during dressing tasks in the dress-up area. She can match basic shapes but has difficulty drawing them from memory. She has difficulty following multiple steps. She has demonstrated some evidence of tactile defensiveness, and difficulty with crossing midline and using trunk rotation. Finally, she has limited in-hand manipulation and fine motor control. Tiffany's general goals included the areas of activities of daily living, fine motor skills for writing, and copying prewriting shapes.

During this day in class, she specifically has requested to finger-paint with her friends. You have the option of working with her in the classroom in the activity of finger-painting.

they are doing client-focused analysis, however. The chosen frame of reference allows the therapist to prioritize which aspects of the task, environment, and context are considered in the analysis with the client. This not only shortens the process of activity analysis completion and uses time and energy efficiently but also allows us to refine our hypotheses regarding client problems and solutions and make the most of the session therapeutically.

For each of the frames of reference discussed above, let us examine how choosing that particular frame of reference might impact the way that you complete a client-focused activity analysis, the aspects of the activity you choose to observe, and the aspects you select to use in therapy (**Table 5-3**). Of primary importance is the consideration between an occupation-based approach and a neuromaturation-based approach. Within any session, you may use one or the other, or both. The decision of approach is made based on the same forms of clinical reasoning discussed. The child's diagnosis, the child and family goals, the setting or context, and the therapy process are all considered in the choice of which approach to take at that moment. In simplistic terms, you need to ask yourself, will you focus on attempting to change the child, trying to "fix" some underlying problem that you have hypothesized is hindering occupational performance, or will you try to adjust or adapt the task, change the environment, or teach the child some alternative way of accomplishing the desired activity?

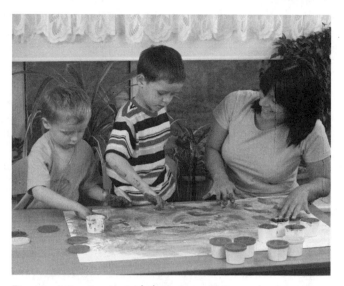

Finger-painting is a typical classroom activity.

In an occupation-based approach, it is the overall performance of the activity that is of primary importance. There is less focus on the individual physiological aspects of the child that may be challenging, and more focus on environmental, contextual, and strategic factors that might affect performance of the activity. Although it is still important to note areas of strength and challenges in the child's inherent ability, this information is not used to directly attempt to change the child. Activity selection, therefore, is based on the chosen frame or frames of reference to elicit the maximal participation in activities related to the child's occupational roles.

When completing a client-focused activity analysis using an occupation-based frame of reference, the therapist should pay particular attention to the child's use of strategies and the development of these strategies; teaching and learning activities of the actual skill in context; and the complexity of the interaction of the child, environment, and task. Less attention is given in these frames of reference to stages of development and inherent physiological characteristics of the child initially, although an underlying assumption in many of these approaches is that the inherent characteristics of the child will change through

Figure 5-1   General Activity Analysis of Finger-Painting

Name of Activity: Finger-painting circles

Description of Activity: While sitting at a table, child will paint circles on large paper using her hands and fingers rather than a paint brush.

Global Demands of the Activity: Demands for this activity include postural control for sitting, reaching for paint, isolating fingers to dip in paint, sufficient motion and strength to reach toward paper, and isolating fingers to form circle. Child must know either how to imitate, copy, or draw a circle, depending on initial direction.

Assumptions About This Activity and Associations Regarding This Activity: This activity is a common childhood activity, usually of younger preschool-age children. The simplicity of the shape may be associated with the young child; however, the actual task of finger-painting can be enjoyed by any age.

Materials Needed for Activity: Finger-paint, paper (preferably large), surface on which to paint, smock.

Space Requirements for This Activity: This activity preferably requires an uncluttered and well-lit space on which to place the paper and paint. It can be done in a small or large room. It could be done on the floor in a prone position or standing, but as considered here, it is done sitting at a table.

Time Requirements for This Activity: The time required to paint a single circle may be seconds to approximately 1 minute; however, the activity can extended if multiple circles are drawn and colored in.

Safety Precautions for This Activity: There is potential for distress if the child has issues with tactile defensiveness or getting messy. Child's finger-paint is nontoxic and safe, although a child who frequently mouths his or her hands and fingers should be watched carefully to avoid unnecessary ingestion of paint.

List all steps for this activity.
Step One: Extend index finger and flex other fingers
Step Two: Dip index finger in paint
Step Three: Place finger on paper
Step Four: Draw circle with paint

Step # 1	Extend index finger and flex other fingers
Sensory input/feedback provided	Proprioceptive input from joints in relation to position of hand
Motor output required	Coordination to bend fingers and thumb while maintaining extension in index finger
Specific muscles and joints used and range of motion required	Index finger extensors, thumb and finger flexors 3–5; adequate extension and flexion to isolate finger
Laterality and crossing midline required	Unilateral activity (can be adapted to be bilateral as well)
Strength required	Minimal strength to maintain flexion and extension of fingers
Endurance required	Minimal endurance required, hand position can be maintained loosely
Position/posture required	Standing or seated
Body awareness required	Minimal body awareness
Mobility required	Minimal
Novelty of the motion/amount of praxis required	Once position reached, no novel movement; child must maintain hand position

Step #2	Dip index finger in paint
Sensory input/feedback provided	Tactile input from paint Visual input to locate cup and guide reach
Motor output required	Accuracy to reach to target of cup Coordination of shoulder movement with isolating index finger
Specific muscles and joints used and range of motion required	Index finger extensors, thumb and finger flexors 3–5; adequate extension and flexion to isolate finger Shoulder flexors to reach to cup; flexion to height of cup required to reach cup
Laterality and crossing midline required	Unilateral reach required
Strength required	Gravity hinders, reaching arm against gravity toward cup No appreciable effect of gravity for fingers
Endurance required	May be several repetitions to get more paint Depending on placement of cup; endurance to lift arm and position hand for several repetitions required
Position/posture required	Standing or seated
Body awareness required	Minimal body awareness required. Knowledge of body in relation to cup for reaching, awareness of hand for positioning when dipping finger and to prevent knocking over cap
Mobility required	No transitional movements required
Novelty of the motion/amount of praxis required	Minimal praxis to position hand with index finger extended

Step #3	Place finger on paper
Sensory input/feedback provided	Tactile cue from paper Visual input to target paper
Motor output required	Shoulder extension to lower arm and accurate target to paper
Specific muscles and joints used and range of motion required	Shoulder extensors and flexors to smoothly lower arm without dropping arm. Minimal range of motion at shoulder
Laterality and crossing midline required	Unilateral
Strength required	Gravity assists to lower arm and motion is not resisted
Endurance required	Minimal endurance
Position/posture required	Standing or seated
Body awareness required	Minimal awareness of body position and hand position in relation to paper
Mobility required	None
Novelty of the motion/amount of praxis required	Lowering arm not a novel task, some planning for placement on paper

(continues)

Figure 5-1   General Activity Analysis of Finger-Painting (continued)

Step #4	Draw circle with paint
Sensory input/feedback provided	Visual feedback of hand on paper to guide shape formation Tactile input from paint and paper
Motor output required	Coordination of eyes and hand to draw shape and for accuracy in shape formation during visual motor output required
Specific muscles and joints used and range of motion required	Index finger extensors, thumb, and finger flexors 3–5; adequate extension and flexion to isolate finger Shoulder flexors, abductors, and rotators
Laterality and crossing midline required	Unilateral; however, crossing midline to draw the shape if it is large may be required
Strength required	Motion is resisted by paper as child presses finger. No appreciable effect of gravity
Endurance required	Endurance to move hand to complete task needed or to hold up arm depending on location of paper
Position/posture required	Standing or seated
Body awareness required	Position in relation to the paper required
Mobility required	Minimal
Novelty of the motion/amount of praxis required	If child is not familiar with drawing shapes or it is new to him or her, planning for forming the shape is required

Cognitive Requirements of This Activity: Minimal sequencing to know when to get paint and then paint on paper. Minimal demands on attention span to follow through on drawing circle.

Perceptual Requirements of This Activity: Depth perception for accurate reach and target to cup, spatial relations to place shape on paper, shape recognition, form and visual closure to complete shape on paper.

Social-Emotional and Psychological Aspects of This Activity: This activity can be structured, as in drawing a specific shape, or less structured, where the child can be creative and draw whatever he or she wants. This activity can be done alone or cooperatively as a group sharing paper or space. It may require taking turns if paint is shared. In free drawing, there is much opportunity for success and productivity.

engagement in occupation (Law et al., 2005; Polatajko & Mandich, 2004).

Activity selection when using the acquisition frame of reference is relatively straightforward. If self-feeding with a spoon is identified in the evaluation process as an area of difficulty, the activity selected for treatment would be a spoon-feeding activity. Although this activity selection is straightforward, the process of activity analysis becomes particularly important here because the activity will be taught by breaking it down into component parts and skills, and helping the child learn to master individual steps and then the whole. Observation of the child doing the activity allows the therapist to determine the specific portions of the task that are difficult; the therapist then either helps the child learn that portion or alters the task to remove the difficulty, allowing the child to be successful.

Because of the nature of the cognitive approaches, therapists using these frames of reference need to be aware

Table 5-2   Clinical Reasoning Regarding Selection of Finger-Painting for Tiffany

Type of Reasoning	Considerations in Determining if Finger-Painting Is Appropriate for Tiffany
Scientific	*Does this activity address the problem I have hypothesized is the issue for this child?* You know from your general activity analysis of finger-painting that this activity can be used to work on the perceptual and fine motor skills that she has trouble with, as well as other areas of motor difficulties for which you have established goals (see the general activity analysis in Figure 5.1 for specific activity demands for finger-painting). This activity could be appropriate to address these goals. *Evidence? Is there any evidence that this activity might be effective?* You are unaware of any specific studies of finger-painting. However, you know from research that clients make greater improvements when they are invested in the activities you use in therapy. You know that some evidence suggests the importance of working with more skilled peers in elevating a child's performance. You also know that if finger-painting is a regular activity in the classroom, then by focusing directly on finger-painting in the classroom, you will not have to be concerned about generalization of skills to the natural environment.
Pragmatic	*In what setting am I practicing? Does that influence my choice of activities in any way? Are there games and activities that I cannot engage in? What materials and resources are available? Do I have the proper space to do this activity safely?* You are in Tiffany's classroom, and you have all the necessary equipment and materials to complete this activity. There is proper space and lighting. This is an educationally related activity that is already occurring in her classroom at this time, and it is therefore one appropriate choice.
Interactive	*What is fun and meaningful for the child? What does this child like and enjoy? In what aspects of the activity is the child most interested?* Tiffany has clearly indicated an interest in this activity. You know that playing with her peers is very important to her. You are not certain which aspects of the activity might be most interesting to her at the moment; but based on your knowledge of Tiffany, you hypothesize it could be the social interaction with her peers. You also know Tiffany's nature and can expect a serious "fight" if you refuse her and try to coax her into doing something else. From past experience, you know her strong-willed nature can lead to power struggles that last 15 minutes or more.
Narrative	*What are the child's roles at home, school, and in the community, and what activities are associated with them? What are the goals identified by the child and the family?* Tiffany's primary roles at this time are daughter, sibling, and student. Although this activity is not a necessary one for any of her current roles, you consider that this activity might be one she could engage in with her older sister or other members of her family. Additionally, you consider that this activity provides you with a fun way to work toward prewriting skills needed for her role as student. During your evaluation process, you determined from the family that they strongly emphasize Tiffany's full inclusion in all school and community events to the best of her ability. Finger-painting is a common childhood and school activity. They find social interaction with her peers to be quite important and stress the importance of her learning socially appropriate behaviors above specific fine motor skills, for example.

(continues)

Table 5-2   Clinical Reasoning Regarding Selection of Finger-Painting for Tiffany (continued)

Ethical	*What are the risks and benefits of the potential therapeutic activity? Am I equipped and trained to select, use, and adapt this type of therapeutic activity?*
	In this situation, no formal training is required to use finger-painting, and there are no serious risks associated with this task. However, in choosing to spend a therapy session in this way, you are using therapy dollars, and you must always choose to spend those therapy dollars wisely. Is this the most effective use of your time at this moment, or would another activity choice be better? If you refuse her request to participate in this activity, how will that influence her cooperation with you in whatever other activity to attempt? Will you get more out of the session if you select the activity that she already wishes to do?
Conditional	*What is the possible future for this child, and does the activity choice help the child toward reaching that possible future?*
	Although, of course, the actual future for Tiffany is unknown, based on your experience with many other similar children and everything you know as a therapist and person, you hypothesize that Tiffany should be able to graduate high school and then perhaps live in a group home and have some form of employment. Although it may not be important in her future to be able to write more than her name, appropriate behaviors and social skills may be key to her ability to get and keep a job. If you had to balance working on specific motor skills or social skills, the social skill issues might be most important in the long term. Tiffany has many years of school ahead of her first, and the ability to demonstrate what has been learned in school often includes being able to write. This activity can be used to focus on both areas at once. You can practice prewriting skills while finger-painting and also work on social interactions with peers at the same time.

that activity selection should be occupation based, allow opportunities for the child to discover and use cognitive strategies, and provide opportunities to process the child's awareness of performance. Activity analysis when using cognitive approaches would focus particular attention to these opportunities and the child's current strategies and approaches to motor skills. During cognitive approaches, activities must be selected that will not only allow the child to practice and learn a variety of cognitive strategies but will also be appealing and motivating for the child. For example, a child with mild motor difficulties may want to learn to jump rope, and the therapist may choose a cognitive approach to help the child learn to jump rope if she or he decides that the child's motor abilities are sufficient to do the task with the proper cognitive sequencing strategies in place. The therapist would select jumping rope as the activity to observe and analyze, and then practice jumping rope using appropriate strategies until the child is able to complete the activity with the strategies independently.

Activity selection in motor learning may be more geared toward providing a task that elicits specific desired motor patterns. When selecting activities from this perspective, the therapist must ensure opportunities for the child to receive both intrinsic and extrinsic feedback on his or her motor performance and opportunities for varied types of practice and repetition. Often, tasks are broken down into smaller parts when using the frame of reference, so detailed sequential analysis of the steps of an activity is important. For example, if the child wishes to be able to bat at a ball in baseball and the therapist believes it is the motor pattern of the swing that is limiting performance, the activity selected in therapy may be a batting game where the child practices the motion of swinging at a target in a variety of ways.

As a reminder, activity selection and analysis with neuromaturation-based frames of reference focus less on the performance outcome and more on the underlying abilities of the child. When using an NDT frame of reference, client-focused analysis of an activity should focus primarily on the motor skills and patterns of the child during the activity. When selecting activities using NDT as the framework, therapists should consider the demands and effects of the activity on the child's postural alignment and control and movement patterns, including transitional movements, reaching, and other functional movement patterns (Schoen & Anderson, 1999). Because therapeutic handling and facilitation by the therapist is a major component of NDT intervention, activities should be selected and designed to allow opportunity for handling, followed by functional practice for the child.

In addition to therapeutic handling techniques, activity selection using this frame of reference might also include specific equipment such as balls, bolsters, and wedges. Although engagement in occupation is the end goal, immediate goals of therapeutic activity usually are targeted toward promoting changes in the child's postural control and alignment and improving quality of movement patterns (Schoen & Anderson, 1999). For example, if the therapist believes that a child's poor postural control is what is limiting his ability to be independent on the toilet, then rather than practice toileting or provide cognitive strategies for toileting, the therapist may choose activities that work on postural control with facilitation, in the belief that improved postural control will lead to improved independence with toileting. The activity chosen in therapy may not look anything like sitting on a toilet, but the demands of the activity chosen will have similar postural demands as toileting. As you can see, in creating this match of activity demands, both general and client-focused activity analyses are critical.

When using the SI frame of reference, therapists focus their attention on the sensory systems of primary importance identified by Ayres (1979, 2005), including the tactile, proprioceptive, and vestibular systems in particular. Client-focused activity analysis includes observations of the child's behavioral responses to sensory aspects of the selected activity, and the chosen activity for observation therefore must be one that offers sensory experiences. Careful attention must be paid to the sensory demands of any potential activity, and a careful match must be made between the child's sensory processing and these sensory demands. In addition, activity selection when using an SI frame of reference should include attention to the child's inner drive. Activities should be sensory rich, not repetitive, and geared toward facilitating an adaptive response and greater abilities in praxis (Kimball, 1999; Parham & Mailloux, 2005). Activity selection should strive for the just right challenge described by Ayres (1979) and the literature so that the child experiences both success and challenge. When using a classic ASI approach, activity selection should occur in an environment that is sensory rich, with varied and safe opportunities to explore sensory experiences on a variety of types of equipment and generate the novelty needed to engage motor planning (Parham & Mailloux, 2005).

What is often confusing to students and novice therapists is that because of the complex nature of activity demands, the same activity can be used in a variety of ways and may be chosen for very different reasons. The same activity can be used with multiple frames of reference. However, the differences are the therapist's immediate goals, the rationale for the selected activity, and the specific activity demands that are emphasized, and then the approach taken to intervention. To illustrate this concept, let us return to Tiffany and make some observations of her completing the activity of finger-painting.

Selecting an Activity for Tiffany

The therapist has decided to use finger-painting as the therapeutic activity. She begins by suggesting that Tiffany gather the materials she needs. When asked what she needs in order to finger-paint, she forgets that she needs her smock, but with reminders, Tiffany runs to the smock bin with a giggle. She is unable to orient the smock to place her arms in and also loses her balance when her shirt is up over her head. She appears uncertain of the steps to the activity and actually sticks her hand in the paint before she has a smock on and the paper is set. She is unable to isolate her individual fingers, instead using her whole arm and hand while painting circles, and she winces and shakes her hand when it contacts the paint. Instead of rotating at her trunk to cross the large paper, Tiffany walks around the entire paper to reach the ends. She attempts to imitate a circle, stating with a smile the verbal cue "around and stop" in imitation of the teacher, and she manages to successfully produce one somewhat recognizable circular shape. She becomes visibly upset when paint splashes onto her arm and immediately asks to wash her hands and arms. When her teacher suggests that she move to an easel to paint with a brush, Tiffany complains of being tired, sits down on the floor, and refuses to participate, humming with her hands over her ears.

Tiffany expressed that she wants to finger-paint. However, when she is led to the table, after getting her smock, she experiences difficulty with maintaining an upright position in sitting, reaching and holding, and finger isolation. The therapist hypothesizes that this could be due to poor postural control, low tone, limited strength, poor endurance, and limited fine motor/manipulative skills. The therapist observes Tiffany using a verbal strategy somewhat successfully to complete a rudimentary circle but notes that Tiffany does not receive any feedback regarding her circle when she completes it. Finally, the therapist observes Tiffany's overresponsiveness to paint on her hands and arms. The therapist hypothesizes that Tiffany may be experiencing a defensive reaction to tactile stimuli and that this may have become increasingly irritating to the point that she can no longer engage in the activity. The result is a behavioral outburst. Given these hypotheses, the therapist decides to consider the activity and the observations she has made from varied perspectives: cognitive, NDT, SI, and acquisitional (**Table 5-4**).

In the situation with Tiffany, the selected activity has been initially unsuccessful. However, the additional knowledge the occupational therapist now has can inform the clinical reasoning process and help the therapist to decide

Table 5-3   Applying Frames of Reference to Activity Selection

Frame of Reference	Activity Analysis and Selection Focus
Acquisition	Activities use teaching and learning methods
	Direct instruction, engagement, and repetition emphasized
	Activities identified as difficult are the actual activities used in therapy
Cognitive	Activities are performed using cognitive strategies to shape successful performance
	Cognitive strategies are generalized through practice and use of the strategies in many different contexts
	Activities are occupation based and allow for real-time feedback related to performance
Motor learning	Activities focus on motor patterns and synergies used by the child
	Practice and repetition with knowledge of performance and results emphasized in all activities
Compensatory	Activities used in therapy are based on activities the child finds difficult
	Child is taught strategies to use during an activity or new ways to perform a modified activity
NDT	Activities focus on postural control, movement patterns, and coordination
	Activities use hands-on facilitation and handling by the therapist and also may use specific types of equipment
SI	Activities need to provide opportunities for child-directed and varied sensory input
	Activities should enable an adaptive response that may then be generalized to other situations
	Activities use particular types of equipment and settings

Learning Activity

Based on what you have now read about Tiffany, which frame of reference would you be most likely to select, and how would you approach the activity of finger-painting in the future? Do you use finger-painting again or avoid it based on her responses? Be explicit in examining which factors are most important in making your decision.

Now consider another activity for Tiffany. Complete a general and a client-focused activity analysis of this activity. What frame or frames of reference influence your activity selection? Be explicit.

Table 5-4   **Comparison of Client-Focused Activity Analysis of Finger-Painting Within Different Frames of Reference**

Frame of Reference	Activity Features[*]	Tiffany's Performance[†]	Application to Use as a Therapeutic Activity
Cognitive	Finger-painting requires an understanding of the sequence of the painting activity, the materials needed, and, in the case of forming shapes or letters, the direct steps or specific motor actions to form those shapes or letters.	Tiffany is uncertain of the materials needed and order of the steps for the activity. Tiffany is attempting to use strategies, including verbal mediation, to draw a circle but does not receive feedback or support on this.	During finger-painting, teach and use cognitive strategies for identifying and remembering steps and sequence of activity and materials needed. Reinforce and give feedback regarding performance of motor task and use of strategy. Follow with the use of the same strategies in similar tasks and activities that do not use finger-paint.
NDT	Finger-painting requires that she maintain an upright posture during painting, that she have adequate reach on and off her base of support, that she has adequate grasp and stroke patterns, and that she can cross midline with trunk rotation to reach all areas of the large paper.	Tiffany has difficulty remaining in an upright seated position. She has difficulty maintaining balance when putting on her smock. She also has difficulty isolating her finger when painting, and she does not cross midline with rotation but instead walks around the paper.	During activities, use therapeutic handling and motor practice in context with facilitation to address trunk strength and rotation when reaching, reaching on and off base of support, and proximal stability with finger isolation. The activity of finger-painting itself may or may not be used. Any activity with those same necessary components will be acceptable.
SI	Finger-painting primarily provides tactile input in terms of the texture and feel of the paint and the temperature of the paint. In addition, this activity requires crossing midline on large paper, bilateral and unilateral hand use, motor planning for forming letters, and planning painting.	Tiffany has difficulty orienting the smock and placing her arms in. She becomes upset when paint touches her hands, but she is unaware of paint on her arms and face without cues. She does not cross midline with rotation but instead walks around paper. Her motor planning for shape and letter formation is poor.	Use deep touch pressure and proprioceptive activities to address tactile sensitivity. Work toward improved tactile discrimination. Modify activities as necessary to change sensory input and demands for participation. Develop and use a variety of activities to address motor planning. It is likely, based on her reaction, that finger-painting may not be used again in the near term until she is better able to tolerate this type of input. Other activities may be selected to work on the goal areas being addressed by finger-painting in this session. Over time, this activity could be attempted again to judge progress.
Acquisitional approach with compensatory strategies	Finger-painting requires maintenance of upright posture, joint mobility and strength to reach, finger isolation, endurance to complete task, vision, and cognitive demands such as sequencing.	Tiffany has decreased endurance for sitting, poor finger isolation, and limited balance when putting on clothes, and she is uncertain of the steps of task and the materials.	During finger-painting, identify and use modifications for seating or position to decrease the demands on her postural control and endurance. Tiffany could finger-paint prone on the floor, standing at an easel, or sitting supported on someone's lap or in a more supportive seat. Create a visual material list or sequence of the activity for Tiffany to use. A tool could be provided for her to use instead of her finger to get the paint, and she could paint using her whole hand if the desired outcome was for her to paint with her peers and engage in classroom activities.

[*]Taken from general activity analysis.
[†]Taken from client observation and specific activity analysis.

quickly whether to adapt the activity and try to get Tiffany to continue, or to rapidly select an alternative activity.

■ CONCLUSION

As a therapist becomes more experienced, he or she is better able to quickly analyze an activity as it relates to a particular child and frame of reference, and make spontaneous activity selections. Certain frames of reference, particularly SI and certain cognitive approaches, promote the use of spontaneous and/or child-led activity within a session. This type of intervention requires the therapist to think quickly to select or create activities that follow the child's lead *and* that remain therapeutic. Once an activity is selected, however, this does not mark the end of the clinical reasoning process or of the use of frames of reference. As Tiffany's case illustrates, just as important, or perhaps sometimes more important, to the therapeutic process is activity adaptation, which will be discussed in Chapter Six.

6

Adapting Play Activities

After reading this chapter the reader will

1. Define and compare the terms "adaptation," "modification," and "grading" in relation to therapeutic activities.

2. Describe considerations for adapting activities based on various frames of reference.

3. Articulate the importance of grading therapeutic activities in developing the "just right challenge."

4. Identify ways to modify the context when planning for playful therapeutic activities.

> *A child loves his play, not because it's easy,*
> *but because it's hard.*
> —Benjamin Spock

Once selected, an activity often must be adapted if it is not the right choice or fit for the child. Perhaps the child is not experiencing the measure of success necessary for him or her to continue without giving up. Or perhaps the activity is so easy that there is no therapeutic benefit for the child. It may be that the therapist is still getting to know the child. Even experienced therapists sometimes choose activities that end up being unsuitable. Sometimes activities that work well one day do not work the next. Perhaps the child is having a difficult day. Children develop and grow quickly and can change dramatically in brief periods of time. What was once difficult may come more easily later on, and vice versa. Just as skills change, interests can vary widely, and motivation levels can differentially affect performance. When these situations arise,

therapists combine activity analysis with their knowledge of the child and the environment to make quick decisions on how best to alter the activity. To maintain the highest level of motivation and therapeutic benefit, therapists are constantly adapting activities during treatment.

■ ACTIVITY ADAPTATION: GRADING AND MODIFICATION

Activity adaptation in occupational therapy includes two processes, grading and modification. Grading is the process of making portions of the activity easier or more difficult based on the client's performance. For example, grading a throwing task for a child could include moving the target closer or farther, making the target larger or smaller, or having the target stationary or moving. Modification of an activity requires altering some aspect of the task to allow a client to perform it. For example, for a child without gross grasp who has full active range of motion in the upper extremity, a painting activity could be modified by using a strapping mechanism to strap a paintbrush to the child's hand. This modification allows the child to paint at an easel like his or her peers. **Table 6-1** describes examples of both forms of adaptation.

Grading

Grading has traditionally been used in occupational therapy practice to "challenge the patient's ability by progressively changing the process, tools, materials, or environment of a given activity to gradually increase or decrease performance demands" (American Occupational

Table 6-1 Examples of Grading and Modification

Grading to Increase Therapeutic Benefit	Modification to Allow Maximal Participation
• Using tongs with more or less resistance to increase or decrease demand on strength	• Using enlarged handles or straps on feeding or writing utensils
• Making a wider or narrower pathway or adding/removing obstacles to navigation for a scooter, wheelchair, or bike	• Using a keyboard (as opposed to writing) to create a story
• Increasing or decreasing the numbers of steps in a sequenced task	• Using stamps instead of crayons to create a picture
• Beginning with some steps already completed	• Extending time for all writing activities
• Reversing or reordering steps of activity	• Using adaptive equipment to hold a paintbrush so a child can paint at an easel
• Increasing/decreasing number and type of cues for a step	• Using a communication device during game/activity to increase social interaction
• Altering communication strategies to be easier or more challenging (e.g., play game using only gestural/nonverbal cues)	• Adapting activities to be done with one hand, one eye, one foot, or different body parts
• Altering the number of individuals involved in a game (play games in pairs or teams)	• Altering a bike so it can be pedaled with the arms rather than the legs
• Altering material availability to encourage sharing	• Completing an activity in a different position from typical
• Increasing or decreasing the time allotted for a task or activity	• Increasing visual contrast so that a child can trace
• Timing an activity that was previously not timed	• Stringing beads on pipe cleaners instead of laces so that a child can do the activity independently
• Using materials that are heavier or lighter	• Altering toys with switch adaptations so that the child may access and play with them independently
• Increasing or decreasing the sensory stimulation provided by an activity	• Changing the rules of a game to allow increased success or participation
• Placing objects to increase or decrease range of motion needed	• Altering playing pieces of commercially available games to enable more independent participation
• Placing things closer or farther away	• Using adaptive tools for writing, coloring, or cutting to increase successful participation
• Altering the manipulation strategy used (increase the challenge level of manipulative games by identifying which finger or fingers the child may use, encouraging the use of dominant or nondominant hand, or both, to increase or decrease the demand)	
• Increasing or decreasing the motion of objects or surfaces to alter motor demands	

Please note for some activity demands, modification and grading ideas may be similar; however the *intent* of the adaptation is what identifies it as either *modification* or *grading*. If the intent is to allow maximal participation in context, then this is a *modification*. If the intent is to increase or decrease the level of demand for therapeutic benefit, then this is considered *grading*.

Therapy Association [AOTA], 1993). Grading is central in achieving the "just right challenge" (Ayres, 1979, 2005). By increasing or decreasing the demands of the activity, grading makes the activity immediately easier or more difficult and therefore potentially more therapeutic. Consequently, grading often occurs multiple times throughout an intervention session as an ongoing process, allowing the child to achieve therapeutic goals.

Pediatric therapists must be ready at a moment's notice to make immediate changes during an activity based on the real-time performance and reactions of the child. These instances are difficult to anticipate, but the therapist's skill during these moments can often "make or break" an intervention session. Activities that are too hard can lead to frustration, anger, tantrums, and refusals to continue to participate. Activities that are too easy can lead to boredom, wandering attention, and eventual refusal to participate. The therapist must skillfully observe the child's reactions and alter activities accordingly to continually motivate the child to engage and meet the next challenge (see Chapter Seven for more details on this process in relation to play).

Activities can be graded to increase or decrease the challenge level in a variety of ways. One of the primary ways that activities are graded is based on the match between a child's ability level and individualized goals, and the demands of the activity itself. The therapist should already understand the demands of the activity through general activity analysis. The therapist combines this knowledge with knowledge of the client gathered through evaluation and ongoing intervention in order to choose which aspect of the activity should be graded (**Figure 6-1**).

Modification

According to the Occupational Therapy Practice Framework (AOTA, 2008) and Dunn, McClain, Brown, and Youngstrom (1998, p. 533), modification is a specific type of occupational therapy intervention defined as "an intervention approach directed at finding ways to revise the current context or activity demands to support performance in the natural setting… [which includes] compensatory techniques, including enhancing some features to provide cues, or reducing other features to reduce distractibility." Activity modification becomes necessary when the given form of the chosen activity is not within the child's current capabilities. Modification of an activity involves changing some aspect of the activity to enable the participation of the client. It is typically used only to make

Figure 6-1   Questions to Ask to Help Problem Solve During Activity Grading

- Was the initial presentation of the activity an appropriate challenge level for the child?
- Has the child been able to perform or engage successfully in this task before?
- Is the child's inability to engage in the activity due to an extenuating or unusual contextual circumstance?
- What aspects of the task are amenable to grading, and are the necessary materials and skills present?
- What aspects of the child's skills and abilities are currently hindering performance, and how can the activity be made easier to allow success? *Or* What aspects of the activity are too easy for the child, and how can the task be made slightly more difficult to create an attainable challenge?
- If the activity cannot be graded, are there alternative activities in which to engage the child?

an activity easier for the client to participate in successfully. Modification may include changes to the context (see Adapting the Activity Context for Play section later in this chapter) or the structure or form of the activity, such as the use of adaptive equipment to perform a task. These modifications are changes made to how the activity is performed in order to enable the child to participate. Modification is used regularly as part of the compensatory frame of reference in circumstances where the child could not participate in the activity otherwise. An example is providing switch access so a child may play with a toy. In this example, the play activity has been modified—that is, the structure or form is different—so the child may then participate in the activity.

Grading and Modifying Activities Using Clinical Reasoning and Frames of Reference

The clinical reasoning process not only impacts activity analysis and selection, as described previously, but also influences our therapeutic choices when grading or modifying activities during intervention (**Figure 6-2**). Scientific reasoning enables us to choose the lens or lenses with which to view the child. When approaching intervention from a particular frame of reference, the therapist often makes choices about how to adapt activities for therapeutic

Figure 6-2   The Process of Utilizing Activity Analysis, Frames of Reference, and Clinical Reasoning in the Intervention Process

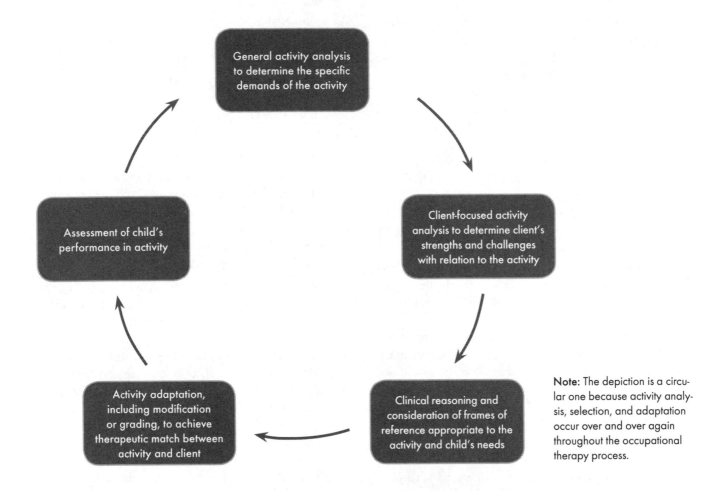

Note: The depiction is a circular one because activity analysis, selection, and adaptation occur over and over again throughout the occupational therapy process.

benefit according to that theoretical framework. Considerations might include whether the frame of reference places more emphasis on modification or grading, what the frame of reference has to say about the different aspects of activity demands, and what the frame of reference identifies as outcomes of therapy. For example, the neurodevelopmental treatment and sensory integration frames of reference place more emphasis on grading aspects of the activity (motor or sensory), with the outcome of intervention being a change in performance skills that leads to a change in participation in a variety of activities. Knowing the tenets of the chosen frames of reference will guide decisions regarding which aspects of the activity are manipulated for therapeutic benefit (**Table 6-2**).

Pragmatic considerations certainly affect the therapist's ability to adapt activities. Available materials, space, time, and other contextual factors influence which aspects

---

Learning Activity

Now consider again the case of Tiffany presented in Chapter Five, and all the information presented so far on frames of reference and activity adaptation. Choose three frames of reference and give specific examples of how you would adapt (either modify or grade) finger-painting for Tiffany according to the principles of that frame of reference.

---

of an activity can be changed and how. Obviously, a modification can only be made if the materials are available and the therapist has the skill to modify the activity. Grading can occur based on what is available in the environment at the moment. Although at times a challenge, meeting pragmatic demands is one of the most rewarding creative endeavors in which occupational therapists engage.

Table 6-2   **Frames of Reference and Activity Adaptation**

Frames of Reference	Activity Adaptation Considerations
Acquisition	Activity is taught and also may be adapted by breaking it down into discrete sequenced steps.
Cognitive	Adaptation (primarily modification) is directed by and occurs with the input of the child as he or she problem solves strategies. Feedback from the performance of an activity may direct the manner in which the activity is adapted (primarily modified).
Motor learning	Activities are adapted to provide continued practice and intrinsic and extrinsic feedback based on the prior performance of the same discrete activity.
Compensatory	Adaptation focuses on modification of the context and activity demands.
Neurodevelopmental treatment	Focus is on grading activities to bring about progressive improvement in the child's motor and postural skills.
Sensory integration	Activity adaptation focuses on grading to provide the right level of challenge to the child. Activity modification may occur to control levels and types of sensory input provided within the activity in order to promote an adaptive response.

Interactive and narrative reasoning are at the heart of establishing and adapting meaningful and playful interactions and activities for pediatric clients. Through this type of reasoning, play schemes and themes are developed and consistently altered to establish and maintain a playful and motivating environment. This reasoning enables therapists to understand the daily routines and situations that the child may encounter and tailor therapeutic activities that best address the demands of those situations. It is also this type of reasoning that helps the therapist grade activities playfully because he or she will have used this type of reasoning to get to know the child and family on a more personal level. Grading activities in a playful manner can often mean the difference between a child coming away from an activity feeling either bored when an activity is too easy or frustrated when it is too hard, and a child feeling able to move forward and try a different activity or a different version of the current activity.

Therapists can use many strategies to address the important social-emotional efficacy aspect of having to change an activity. Therapeutic use of self (see Chapter Four) is an important tool in this process. For example, the occupational therapist may take the blame for making an activity too easy or too hard. Statements like "Oh my, I put that way too high didn't I? I can barely reach it. Let me fix it and then we can try again" or "Wow, I made that as wide as a river, who can jump a whole river? Not me. I better make it smaller" can go a long way toward framing a child's perspective positively. Competition, if a child can handle it, can be useful when upgrading an activity. A theme that you know is a child's favorite and that is easily changed to make the level easier or harder can be helpful in easing any anxiety the child might feel if he or she cannot accomplish a task as it was originally presented. Interactive and narrative reasoning provide important information about what play themes may be fun and meaningful to the child. Further detailed play applications are provided in Chapters Seven and Eight.

Ethical reasoning allows us to consider what will benefit the child and pose the least risk. Ethical reasoning is important when considering adaptation, especially in certain settings. If a child would benefit more from being able to participate with a modification, then clearly the emphasis should be placed on modifying the activity for maximal participation, at least until the child has enough skills to participate otherwise. In some cases, depending on client factors, diagnosis, or other physical considerations, it may be apparent that the child cannot participate in an activity without modifications. It is in these situations that we as occupational therapists can play an important role in using our expertise in activity analysis to find ways to modify aspects of the task so that the child may engage and participate in it.

■ ADAPTING THE ACTIVITY CONTEXT FOR PLAY

Because the activity is interconnected with the physical, social, and cultural environment in which it occurs, contextual adaptations must also be considered for their impact on adapting activities for play. Given this book's particular focus on play and in preparation for the next two chapters' focus on play adaptations, we highlight specific considerations of contextual adaptations for promoting play.

By structuring the environment, the therapist can use fewer directions to "do this" and fewer rules to limit behavior ("no _____") so that the child experiences greater relative internal control to play. The occupational therapist may target the environment through direct therapy to facilitate play during therapy, or in consultation and advocacy with others to adapt the natural daily living environments to promote the child's play. Occupational therapists manage the environment for maximal function in daily activities and maximal participation in therapeutic activities (Dunning, 1972; McEwen, 1990). The physical setting, people, and materials must be selected, adapted, and structured to match the client's needs. The child must have safe, adequate, and flexible space in which play can occur and his or her goals can be addressed. The space should be arranged to allow the child easy access to those materials that the therapist wants the child to explore. Likewise, materials that require supervision or that limit play may be placed out of reach but should be easily accessible by the therapist when needed. The environment should allow for adaptation to move materials to create and adapt for play. The environment sends cues to the child about whether play is accepted in this environment and what kind of play can occur (Frost, Shin, & Jacobs, 1998).

Environmental Adaptations

Adapting natural environments is one way of facilitating play in children (Ideishi, Ideishi, Gandhi, & Yuen, 2006). The environment is modified through providing expert consultation and/or advocacy with others to promote the child's participation in play activities (Canadian Association of Occupational Therapists, 1996). Examples include

assisting parents with managing the home play objects and spaces (Pierce, 2000), instructing parents in how to make inexpensive toys (Esdaile & Sanderson, 1987), adjusting heights and surfaces in a playground for children with physical disabilities (Stout, 1988), and collaborating or advocating for other changes to physical space, materials, or playmates (Rigby & Huggins, 2003; Rigby & Rodger, 2006). Environmental adaptations can be especially important for children with visual impairments (Retting, 1994) and with physical disabilities, particularly mobility limitations (Skar, 2002). Environmental adaptations ensure that children have an environment in which to play (AOTA, 2007). For an in-depth view of home and community environmental interventions to promote play for children, the reader is referred to Letts, Rigby, and Stewart (2003) and Rodger and Ziviani (2006). This book will highlight adapting and structuring the environment in which therapy occurs.

Safety

The environment must be safe, comfortable, and interesting for the child and others who may be present (Baranek, Reinhartsen, & Wannamaker, 2001; Lally & Stewart, 1990; Lane & Mistrett, 2008; Skard & Bundy, 2008). The child and caregiver should feel safe and relaxed to enable freedom to explore and take risks. The environment must be clean and sanitary. Supplies and strategies for ensuring sanitation between and during sessions must be available. Institutional policies and procedures to ensure health should be developed and followed. The environment should be safeguarded from potential dangers. For example, the occupational therapist must guard against potential injury from tripping/falling hazards, electrical equipment and outlets, sharp items, toxic materials, and small objects on which the child can choke. This may involve altering the environment itself or being prepared to intervene to protect the child. The therapist may use such opportunities to help the child learn about safety in the environment, such as cars in parking lots or children swinging on the playground. Basic first aid supplies should be available to ensure appropriate assistance if an injury occurs. Anticipating potential hazards in the environment allows the occupational therapist to be ready to respond immediately in an effective and sympathetic manner if necessary.

Natural Environment

The therapist may start in the typical environment where the child is, such as home and school. However, the occupational therapist may want to consider other common environments, such as parks and fast-food restaurants, that the family may not have used because of challenges with physical access or concerns about the child's impulsiveness (Hinojosa & Kramer, 2008). A diversity of environments can be important for the child's social interaction and community inclusion. Ideishi et al. (2006) and Miller & Kuhaneck (2008) recommend outdoor environments for play because of their large space, flexibility, and unstructured social agenda. In natural environments, the occupational therapist generally has less control over the environment than in a clinic and must be ready to adapt the environment and treatment activities. When venturing into new environments, more planning and onsite clinical reasoning are required to ensure the client's safety and success.

Social Environment: Peers and Other Social Groups

Treatment planning also considers aspects of the social environment that support or impede play (Humphry & Wakeford, 2006; Rigby & Huggins, 2003; Sturgess, 2003). First, the occupational therapist, through therapeutic use of self, creates a therapeutic social environment that promotes play (see Chapter Four). Second, the occupational therapist must consider who else is involved in sessions and the nature of their involvement. As primary play partners, family members may be included in therapy sessions. Peers may be primary play partners or may be desired future play partners. The therapist may want to consider having peers present to support a playful environment and/or to build play skills (Baranek et al., 2001; Florey & Greene, 2008). The occupational therapist may also need to help family members and peers adapt their strategies to create a playful experience (Hinojosa & Kramer, 2008; Lally & Stewart, 1990; Lane & Mistrett, 2008; Skard & Bundy, 2008).

Just like new occupational therapists, parents and peers may need assistance to determine how much direction to give and how much control to exert, in order to allow the child to have a balance of freedom and structure to play. Family and peers may need to recognize and respond to small initiations or limited play interests to reinforce and build on the child's efforts. The occupational therapist may note, "Did you see/hear how the child did _____ to show _____?" Helping other players to facilitate play involves teaching them the same particular skills that the therapist is using to help the child play. By explaining why he or she is doing what he or she is doing, by modeling these strategies, by coaching and encouraging the family member or peer, and by noting the child's actual or potential response, the occupational therapist helps the family and peers develop skills for playing with the particular child. By creating a match between players instead of focusing on the child with the disability, the occupational therapist promotes play, especially social play.

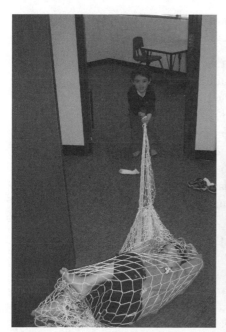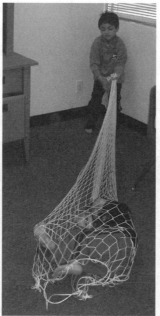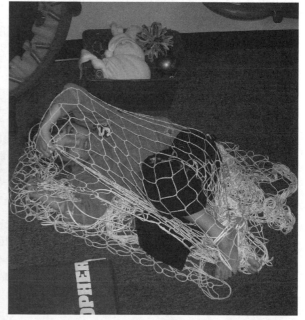

Play can be promoted by including other social play partners. Two brothers work on cooperative play by taking turns being lion and lion catcher.

Materials

Based on an evaluation of what the child can do and what the child needs or wants to do with materials, the occupational therapist determines which and how many materials to have available for use (**Table 6-3**). A general activity analysis provides the characteristics, and the occupational therapist matches these to the individual client. The materials must be matched with the child's interests and abilities (Rigby & Huggins, 2003). There must be enough materials to enable the child to make choices (Lally & Stewart, 1990) and enough variety to build the child's skills (Florey & Greene, 2008). However, there should not be so many materials that social interaction is discouraged (Frost et al., 1998) or that the child becomes overstimulated. The occupational therapist selects and sets up materials that promote play and removes materials that interfere with play (Florey & Greene, 2008; Hinojosa & Kramer, 2008). Florey and Greene (2008) recommended setting up activities in advance for children with behavioral and emotional problems who may have trouble waiting and focusing during set-up. For another child, the therapist may opt to remove a particular object on which the child is focused that cannot be reframed as play or that causes anxiety or negative behaviors.

The occupational therapist carefully considers the properties of materials (Knox, 1993) and how they might be used (Ferland, 2005; Gibson, 1988) through general activity analysis. Based on this knowledge, the occupational therapist considers the materials that are available in relation to the client's interests and therapeutic goals. With creative thought, the occupational therapist can utilize the same physical materials in dramatically different play activities to address the therapeutic needs of diverse clients.

Learning Activity

Develop your skills for creative use of materials in developing therapeutic play activities for individual clients by completing the form in **Appendix 6-1**.

To promote play, the materials should invite the child to participate actively. The materials may be appealing because of their esthetic qualities (Lane & Mistrett, 2008) or because of the child's particular interest. Bright colors are usually appealing (Blanche, 2008; Deitz & Swinth, 2008). A toy is also appealing if it is responsive to the child's actions, such as making a noise or action when the child interacts with it (Blanche, 2008; Deitz & Swinth,

---

Table 6-3   Considerations of Materials for Play in Pediatric Occupational Therapy

Number of objects
- Choice
- Variety
- Arousal level

Type of objects
- Interest
- Aesthetics—bright colors
- React to child's actions (i.e., cause and effect)
- Sensory properties
- Flexibility and variability
- Structure
- Presence in typical environment
- Adaptable/adjustable
- Safety
- Durability
- Age appropriateness (developmental, chronological)
- Novelty
- Social play options
- Interesting to peers
- Potential to address therapeutic needs/goals

2008). Universal design advocates recommend toys with multisensory and multimodal experiences that appeal to a variety of children with and without disabilities (Lane & Mistrett, 2008) and have developed a tool to guide people in selecting toys that meet this criterion (Ruffino, Mistrett, Tomita, & Hajare, 2006; Universal Design for Play Project, 2005) (**Table 6-4**). Generally, flexible features allow for more creative play possibilities, without clear right and wrong ways, and thus are more motivating for a variety of children (Blanche, 2008; Lane & Mistrett, 2008). Toys and materials that can be used in a wide variety of ways include play-dough, water, bubbles, dolls, cups, cars, sand, and swinging (Blanche, 2008). However, some children can become disorganized and distracted by too many options and may need more structure to clarify what to do with a toy (Lane & Mistrett, 2008). A toy must be easy enough to use that it is fun to play with (Blanche, 2008; Lane & Mistrett, 2008).

Table 6-4   Features of Universal Design for Toys

- The toy is appealing.
- How to play with the toy is clear.
- The toy is easy to use.
- The toy is adjustable.
- The toy promotes development.
- The toy can be played with in different ways.

From Universal Design for Play Project (2005). Complete Universal Design for Play Tool available freely online at the Let's Play Web site: *http://letsplay.buffalo.edu/UD/udp_tool.htm*

Selecting and adapting materials for play that also address therapeutic goals requires careful thought. Clinical environments are full of therapeutic materials whose intended use often is not playful (Blanche, 2008). Using toys or props related to favorite television shows, movies, or books can help to incorporate the child's interests into the activity. Florey and Greene (2008) recommended using crafts and games to which the children are otherwise commonly exposed because this allows the child to build skills for activities in which they can participate outside therapy. Selecting commonly available toys accessible to children with disabilities is important (Lane & Mistrett, 2008). However, many commonly available toys may not be of interest to or accessible to children with disabilities. Toys can be modified with adaptive devices such as switches, enlarged handles, or changes in positioning to increase access (Blanche, 2008; Bracegirdle, 1992; Deitz & Swinth, 2008; Ferland, 2005; Hinojosa & Kramer, 2008; Knox, 1993; O'Brien et al., 1998; Williams & Matesi, 1988).

Occupational therapists may also identify alternative, playful ways of using toys and objects. Even common toys or household objects may be used in playful ways (Hinojosa & Kramer, 2008). Certain physical characteristics must be considered. For example, heavy toys may help provide stability for a child with tremors, or feedback in a child with poor kinesthetic awareness. Sometimes, toys and objects are not even needed in play activities because the therapist and child can use their bodies and ideas to invent sensorimotor or pretend games (Hinojosa & Kramer, 2008).

Various other features of materials also should be considered when selecting materials in pediatric occupational therapy. Novelty in materials or their use can be exciting and promote play (Parham, 1992). Safety, durability, and age appropriateness should also be considered (Blanche, 2008), as well as availability and interest for peers. Determining if a toy is safe and durable for a child involves a realistic consideration of what the child may do with the toy. Will the child use the toy in its intended way? How much force may be used considering the child's kinesthetic deficits, frustration tolerance, anger management, and so on? Will the child try to mouth it, break it open, stand on it, or throw it? Age appropriateness involves considerations of both the child's developmental and chronological age. Ideally, materials are appropriate for the child's chronological age because this will help the child be included in the general community. However, if a child's developmental age is significantly lower than his or her chronological age, he or she may not have the interest or ability to engage in age-appropriate play activities. In these cases, the occupational therapist may consider activities that promote a higher play stage (Lane & Mistrett, 2008); consider computer-based activities, which are often interesting to a wide age range of children (Deitz & Swinth, 2008), or consider how to adapt activities to address developmental and chronological age needs.

Learning Activity

Consider a commercially available toy. Using the general activity analysis form, complete a quick general analysis as a guide of how the toy or game would be played with traditionally. Once you have finished, describe at least five ways this toy or game can be adapted (modified or graded) to be used therapeutically.

Because children are part of a social context and because social play is often a goal for children with disabilities, the social properties of the materials are also important. Based on the general activity analysis, the occupational therapist considers how well the properties of the materials are suited for social play (Baranek et al., 2001; Quilitch & Risley, 1973). The availability of, and interest in, play materials among the child's playmates must be considered. For example, what are the preferred activities of children of this age and gender? Are computer games available in this child's everyday context? Is there safe playground equipment available? If materials are not available, the occupational therapist may consult with clients to determine ways to secure such materials. If the child wants to play with materials that are not of interest to other children, the occupational therapist may use these materials but in new ways to bridge the gap between the child and peers.

For example, a child who likes to hold a favorite toy might learn to play catch or tag with that toy with another child or other children. The occupational therapist may use materials of interest to the child in combination with materials that are of interest to the child's peers. For example, a child interested in DVD cases might learn to transport them in a wagon or give them a ride on toy cars. Toys take on emotional properties in addition to their physical ones and can bridge critical gaps between a child and peers and between home and the social world (Kibele, 2008).

■ CONCLUSION

Adapting activities is an essential part of being an effective occupational therapist. Activities may be modified to increase participation or graded to promote optimal therapeutic benefit. Based on activity analysis, occupational therapists use complex clinical reasoning to determine what aspects of the activities and the context to adapt and in what way. Although some adaptations can be planned in advance, many must be determined quickly in the moment of therapy sessions. With a strong knowledge of activity analysis, occupational therapists are uniquely equipped to adapt activities spontaneously in the midst of intervention. This book provides the underlying knowledge and learning strategies to develop this skill; however, you must refine this skill through ongoing practice and mentorship. Next, we apply this knowledge and your developing skill to the selection and adaptation of activities to create *play*.

Appendix 6-1

Learning Activity on Creative Use of Same Materials for Different Clients

Occupational therapists often use the same materials in a variety of different creative and playful ways to address the needs of various clients. Given these commonly available items—large ball, small ball, bucket, bean bag, clothespins, and paper—for each client, consider which frame(s) of reference you would use. Develop two different therapeutic activities both that meet the child's needs and that the child is likely to experience as play. The same activity may be adapted for different clients. The following form can also be found online at *www.jbpub.com*.

Child	Activity 1	Activity 2
Joshua is a 6-year-old with autism and low tone who lacks in-hand manipulation skills. This results in functional difficulty with writing within lined paper, buttoning, and zipping a jacket, which are his goals. His primary interest is outer space.	Frame(s) of Reference: Activity Selected: Adaptations:	Frame(s) of Reference: Activity Selected: Adaptations:
Connor is a 3-year-old boy with Down syndrome who has difficulty using two hands together and predominantly uses a gross palmar grasp prehension pattern. He has a generally low arousal level and lacks interest in fine motor activities but likes to hold animal toys and people figures.	Frame(s) of Reference: Activity Selected: Adaptations:	Frame(s) of Reference: Activity Selected: Adaptations:

Child	Activity 1	Activity 2
Stephanie is an 8-year-old with average cognitive skills, bipolar disorder, and a learning disability. She was referred for slow, difficult, illegible, and large writing (due to poor in-hand manipulation skills) and difficulties with bilateral activities such as cutting, opening food packages, and managing buttons/zippers. She often cries when she makes mistakes and then refuses to do the rest of the activity. She generally prefers to play with toddler-age toys and games.	Frame(s) of Reference: Activity Selected: Adaptations:	Frame(s) of Reference: Activity Selected: Adaptations:
Max is a 14-year-old with mild right hemiplegic cerebral palsy and mild cognitive delays. He is very interested in sports and knows about different players and teams. His writing is very slow, large, and difficult to read. He is learning to type but has difficulty keeping his fingers on the correct keys and individually controlling finger movements to type the correct letter. He says he wants to do his own work but gets very frustrated and does not want to practice writing or typing. He follows your directions but never seems very interested in fine motor activities. You are Max's school occupational therapist.	Frame(s) of Reference: Activity Selected: Adaptations:	Frame(s) of Reference: Activity Selected: Adaptations:

Child	Activity 1	Activity 2
Austin is a 5-year-old boy with average cognitive skills who is fully included in a regular kindergarten. He is generally interested in whatever the other boys in his class are doing. He was born with structural anomalies and has had several surgeries. Currently, each hand has a thumb (no IP joint) and two other short fingers with limited range of motion in the IP joints. He can put on and take off T-shirts and pants with elastic-banded waist. He cannot put on and take off shoes, socks, and jackets or manage any type of clothing fasteners. He wants to dress and undress by himself.	Frame(s) of Reference: Activity Selected: Adaptations:	Frame(s) of Reference: Activity Selected: Adaptations:
Emily is a 20-month-old with spastic cerebral palsy. She has difficulty reaching toys (under- and overshooting) and has difficulty releasing in desired locations, such as into a container. She prefers social play rather than object play.	Frame(s) of Reference: Activity Selected: Adaptations:	Frame(s) of Reference: Activity Selected: Adaptations:

7

Creating Therapeutic Play Activities

After reading this chapter the reader will

1. Explain how to use activity analysis to adapt common daily activities that the child is experiencing as "work" into playful therapeutic activities.

2. Describe why an occupational therapist must be ready to alter a treatment plan and how this clinical reasoning promotes play.

> *Life must be lived as play.*
> —Plato

A young client may pick up a toy, smile, explore it, and hand it to the occupational therapist. From here, the occupational therapist can suggest a playful way of holding or placing the toy to address therapeutic goals. An older child may reach for a rope offered by the occupational therapist and respond, "Hey, I'm Spider-Man!" From here, the occupational therapist and client build a story line around this idea, with the occupational therapist suggesting materials or actions to work on therapeutic goals that are consistent with this story line. This is the ideal, and it is a beautiful, wondrous process when it occurs.

Unfortunately, the reality is that many of our clients do not possess such a playful approach, the ability to contribute their own play ideas, or the ability to easily adapt their play ideas with therapeutic goals. They find a range of activities difficult, challenging, or otherwise frustrating. They often avoid the very types of activities that would be most therapeutic for them. This is why they need occupational therapy.

For these children, the occupational therapist must not only become skilled in playing (see Chapter Four) but also develop skill in creating playful activities. The occupational therapist must possess a strong knowledge of both activity analysis and play, in addition to knowledge of self and the child. Based on this knowledge, the occupational therapist conducts client-focused activity analysis and ongoing assessment that provide the individualized knowledge necessary for creating activities that are playful for an individual child. This clinical reasoning process is reflected in the treatment plan (**Appendix 7-1**, also available online at *www.jbpub.com*) and in ongoing adaptations to the plan. This chapter applies the information gained from Chapters Five and Six, demonstrating the clinical reasoning process involved in making and adapting therapeutic activities into play for the pediatric client.

■ MAKING THERAPEUTIC WORK INTO PLAY

Based on evaluation and activity analysis, the occupational therapist is equipped with the knowledge necessary to create playful work activities. The occupational therapist integrates the knowledge about what the child likes (materials, themes) with knowledge about what the child needs to do. The occupational therapist then combines elements of both into a unique therapeutic activity that the child enjoys. Children with and without disabilities report that they like to participate in activities in which they can have fun and feel success with challenges (Heah, Case, McGuire, & Law, 2007; Miller & Kuhaneck, 2008). The occupational therapist grades and modifies each activity to match the individual client's interests and needs. The work activity is

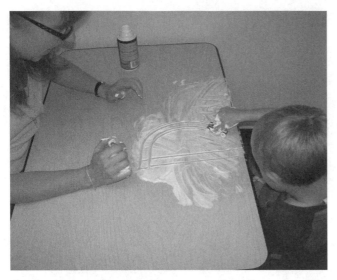

Combining a work activity like writing with a play activity like driving a toy car in shaving cream can make the work more playful for the child.

reframed into a play activity (Spitzer, 2003b, 2004, 2008). In this way, the child engages in work that feels like play.

Transforming the work of daily life and therapy into play in which children want to participate is a core challenge for and skill of the pediatric occupational therapist. Without play, the child can be resistive and even oppositional. But when therapeutic work is transformed into play by a skillful therapist, it seems natural and playful. Ironically, developing and using this skill takes serious work (clinical reasoning). We hope to explicate this process so you have a clear vision of how to make therapy playful and of the possibilities for play in the work of both therapist and client.

Infusing Play into Self-Care

As children develop, they are expected to become more independent in self-care and to tolerate self-care activities as a part of basic hygiene and as members of their social communities. For children with disabilities, self-care activities

---

Eastlyn and Dressing

Eastlyn was a 4-year-old with autism and limited communication skills. She had been receiving occupational therapy for a few months and was making consistent progress. Her mother asked the occupational therapist for help getting Eastlyn ready for an upcoming family trip to snow country. Her mother was concerned that Eastlyn would not be able to participate because she had not been able to get Eastlyn to tolerate wearing even socks or a jacket. Eastlyn also refused all other cold-weather clothes such as boots, mittens, heavy pants, and hat. The occupational therapist identified that Eastlyn's resistance was due to both her preference for structure and routine and her sensory modulation deficits. If Eastlyn could not tolerate appropriate clothing, given the cold climate for their vacation, her health would be jeopardized, or she would have to be inside all day with one parent while her brothers play outside with the other parent.

Eastlyn's mother wanted her to be included as part of the family. In preparation, her mother repeatedly brought out all the cold-weather clothes and had the whole family dress up, but Eastlyn was the only one to resist. It was getting closer to the trip, and Eastlyn was not getting any more comfortable with cold-weather dressing. The occupational therapist asked Eastlyn's mother to bring in these cold-weather clothes. The occupational therapist wanted Eastlyn (1) to have positive feelings about the clothes so that she would be more willing to wear them and (2) to have the proprioceptive-vestibular input that would help make the unfamiliar clothing textures more tolerable.

The occupational therapist planned to combine what Eastlyn needed to do (the winter clothes) with a playful sensory-motor activity that Eastlyn had consistently enjoyed. This play activity consisted of Eastlyn sitting in a swing, climbing backward up a ramp, lifting her feet to swing down the "mountain," and kicking a therapy ball placed on the floor. Eastlyn loved seeing the ball fly to the other end of the room. To add in the clothes, the occupational therapist decided to put them on the ball, telling Eastlyn they were going to "dress" the ball. The therapist asked Eastlyn which item to place next, eventually making a large pile of clothing on and around the ball. After the first time, when the clothing flew all over, Eastlyn laughed and became very interested, directing the therapist in which item to put next. After a few times, the occupational therapist announced that it was "Eastlyn's turn to get dressed." The occupational therapist gave her an option between two items, and Eastlyn picked a jumpsuit. Eastlyn allowed the therapist to help her put it on and then got back on the swing to continue the game. After a few times, the occupational therapist would suggest another item to wear, always giving Eastlyn a choice. They added mittens, a hat, boots, and a scarf until Eastlyn was covered in winter clothing. The occupational therapist also took pictures, which were given to her family to review and discuss how fun it was to get dressed up for the snow. After this one session, Eastlyn was able to tolerate and practice snow dressing with her family at home and wear adequate cold-weather clothing to play in the snow on their family vacation.

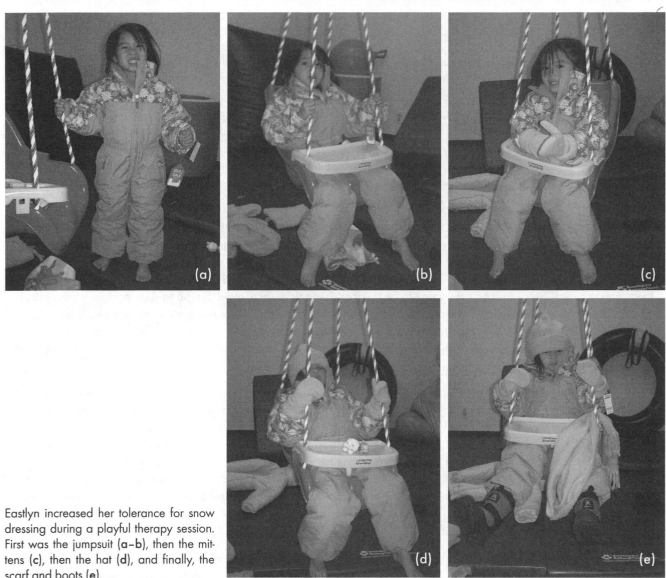

Eastlyn increased her tolerance for snow dressing during a playful therapy session. First was the jumpsuit (**a–b**), then the mittens (**c**), then the hat (**d**), and finally, the scarf and boots (**e**).

Learning Activity

Considering the case of Eastlyn, how could you address the work of dressing differently using play?

---

may be perceived as more work than play. The activities may be physically difficult, or they may be uncomfortable or painful because of sensory sensitivities. Occupational therapists may work on self-care skills or underlying abilities (motor control, bilateral coordination, sensory modulation, etc.) or make modifications that make self-care easier. A playful approach of transforming self-care activities into play can also be used to build skills, to grade therapeutic challenge, and to increase the child's motivation to participate in therapy and in daily life. Case examples on

dressing (Eastlyn), toileting (Devon), and bathing (Lucas) are presented to help the reader visualize how play might be used in therapeutic sessions related to self-care goals.

Other ways of making self-care playful include dressing weighted animals and dolls, performing self-care routines with dolls or stuffed animals, helping a younger sibling with self-care, using a knife and fork to cut french fries or other unusual items, "tying-up" people or toys to practice tying shoelaces, tying string "legs" onto a paper octopus body, tying shoelaces in steps with a pirate story (Steese, 2009), and tying bows on a doll's hair or "gifts."

Infusing Play into Writing

One of the most common reasons children are referred to occupational therapy is for help with writing. Some children have trouble learning to write. Some have difficulty

Devon and Toileting

Devon was a 5-year-old with developmental delays and sensory modulation deficits. He was receiving school occupational therapy services. His preschool teacher was very concerned because Devon refused to go near the bathroom, let alone go in. Generally, he was very compliant and liked to help and please adults, but he became very upset when the staff insisted he use the bathroom. Occasionally, he had accidents and wet his clothing. He was very upset by this but still refused to go into the restroom. Next school year, in kindergarten, the days would be even longer, and Devon's refusal to use the restroom at school would likely interfere more with his educational program. His mother reported that he was independent with toileting at home but refused to use public restrooms in the community. The occupational therapist determined that Devon's resistance to toileting at school was likely due to his sensitivities to sound, because the school restroom had old, loud plumbing that echoed in its large, tiled space.

The occupational therapist decided to schedule her sessions with Devon first thing in the morning, when the routine was for the class to use the restroom. First, she offered Devon interesting fine motor games to play with outside the restroom door. This succeeded in getting Devon out from under the staircase where he liked to wait, and next to the restroom as he waited for the other children. Once he was comfortable enough that he could really enjoy the toys, the occupational therapist then told Devon that he was going to be the restroom helper, and it was his job to push open the heavy door into the restroom. He was initially hesitant; the occupational therapist modeled opening the door first, and then did it together with him until he could do it on his own. In this way, the occupational therapist provided a way for Devon to take two steps into the restroom at a time when it was at its quietest (as the first student in) and get heavy proprioceptive input to modulate his sensory sensitivities and in a role that he enjoyed.

Getting Devon into the restroom for increasing lengths of time was the next step. To prepare, the occupational therapist began to bring toys that could be washed off in the sink. Then she brought soap foam and other substances to put on the toys and suggested to Devon that they give the toys a shower and dry them off in the restroom. First, it was only one toy, and then Devon was able to spend most of the time giving the toys a "shower." Then the therapist had him end by washing his hands. Later, they took the toys to "look in" the toilet stalls. By this time, on the days the occupational therapist was not there, he was consistently coming in with the class and washing his hands during toileting time. When his occupational therapist was transferred to another school, Devon was not yet toileting at school but was well on his way toward that goal.

Learning Activity

Considering the case of Devon, how could you address the work of toileting differently using play?

---

with forming letters correctly or legibly. Others have trouble with speed or sustaining endurance for writing assignments. Although many of these children may want to write better, easier, and faster, they often hate the current overwhelming difficulty of writing and resist it or refuse to *work* on it. In addition to working on underlying foundational components of writing, sometimes occupational therapists need to work with children on writing to develop these skills. In general, children tend to perceive writing as a work activity (Wing, 1995). Making fun from the work of writing is quite a challenge. Here we provide a number of examples of adaptations we have used to make writing more like play:

- Use different materials (soap foam, clay, markers, sand tray, paintbrush dipped in water with a chalkboard, body crayons to make "tattoos," etc.)
- Draw shapes and simple pictures first to get better visual-motor skill for using a pencil
- Play tic-tac-toe with different letters or words instead of Xs and Os
- Play hangman
- Guess the word (write dictated spelled words)
- Write meaningful words that are:
  - About the child's interests (car brands, foods, etc.)
  - About an upcoming event/holiday
  - Funny or socially "inappropriate" by adult standards (**Table 7-1**)
  - Silly made-up words (Many children find it fun to try and sound out words from random letters or hear the therapist do so. The therapist and child can even guess/make up a meaning for the "words.")

Lucas and Bathing

Lucas was a 9-year-old with mild mental retardation, ADHD, and bipolar disorder. He seemed very aware that other children were able to do more than he was and did not like anything that made him feel like he stood out from other children his age. His parents wanted Lucas to be able to bathe himself adequately just like his younger brother was able to do. Lucas was able to get in and out of the shower and turn the water on and off, but he barely wiped soap or a wash cloth on his body, finishing in 30 seconds without completely cleaning himself. When his parents gave him any directions or assistance, he became so angry that he stopped and refused to do any more. If they insisted, his negative behaviors would escalate into yelling, kicking, hitting, and throwing. They had tried a visual list of what to do, but this did not help either. After evaluating Lucas, the occupational therapist determined that Lucas' difficulties in bathing were due to sensitivity to touch, postural instability, poor sequencing, an impulsive and inattentive behavioral pattern, and discomfort with being helped.

Part of their sessions focused on sensory processing and postural control to build underlying foundations for bathing, but Lucas also needed to establish an effective bathing routine. The occupational therapist suggested a "shower" obstacle course with a pretend bathroom, shower, soap, and water. Lucas liked the idea of a new game to play. The occupational therapist guided Lucas to establish rules together, starting from head to toe to make sure that all body parts were "washed" and counting to 10 for each body part to make sure it was washed completely. Lucas helped set up various obstacle courses with each step being a different part of the body to "wash." Lucas especially loved having the occupational therapist take a turn so that he could help her follow the rules (to remember what to do next and be sure she was thorough). In this way, showering was not a battle, but a fun play activity to which Lucas looked forward.

Learning Activity

Considering the case of Lucas, how could you address the work of bathing differently using play?

- Incorporate writing into a play theme:
  - Secret messages to pirates about hidden treasure
  - Notes to leave in hidden places for monsters or ghosts
  - Banners or signs to use in "presentations" such as for a circus, store, etc.
  - Written score in a game with points (or make points up)
  - Rules for an activity
  - Board game with direction cards or written directions
  - Card game with letters, numbers, or words to pick and write
- Write a list of activities the child wants to do or has done
- Make a book about a topic that interests the child:
  - Occupational therapy memories—a picture and caption from each session
  - Jokes
  - Comic/cartoon—draw pictures or use stickers and then make balloons to write in the character comments
  - Favorite subjects such as cars, super heroes, planets, etc.
- Write a letter or word at the end of each pass through an obstacle course or scooter board path
- Keep a graph for the child to record his or her own performance on writing activities to track increasing performance and try to beat his or her previous score (points for amount of writing, speed, neatness, etc.)
- Make up own *MAD LIBS*
- Write a letter to someone real or made up
- Make a list of toys the child wants to get from a catalog
- Combine writing with another favorite interest:
  - For a child interested in geography, make a map of the country with names of all the states written
  - For a child interested in super heroes, when letters do not turn out well, put bad letters in "jail" (draw a square around them and put vertical lines through)
  - For a child interested in a particular character or object, use an appropriate colored pencil to do "_____ writing" such as red for "Spider-Man" writing, black for "Darth Vader" writing, blue for "Cookie Monster" writing, etc.
- Make a label for a food product (e.g., root-beer bottle, soda can, candy bar, cereal box, etc.)

For children learning the prewriting skills of drawing lines and simple shapes, some of the above-listed ideas can be graded for prewriting skills as well. However, you may

Table 7-1   Examples of Words Children May Find More Interesting to Write

barf	gag	poop	spit	wahoo
belch	gas	potty	splat	wart
blah	gooey	pow	stinky	whoop
blast	gross	pus	toilet	yahoo
bonkers	horrifying	quack	trash	yawn
boogers	jabber	sewer	turd	yelp
burp	jeepers	slime	underpants	yuck
butt	jolt	slurp	vapor	zap
crash	ka-boom	smelly	venom	zany
crazy	magic	snarled	vermin	zillion
dodo	maniac	sneeze	vex	zip
fart	ooze	snore	vomit	zoom
flush	pee	snot	wacky	

Note: These words are presented as examples of what some children may prefer to write. They should be used with caution, in consideration of the child's sociocultural environment.

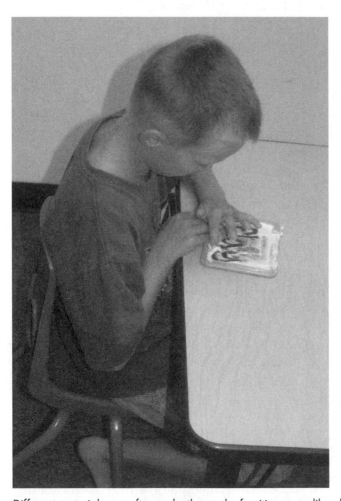 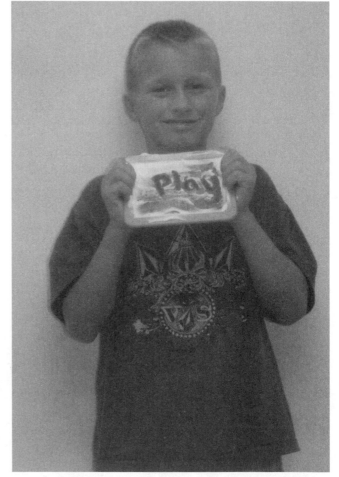

Different materials can often make the work of writing more like play.

Toni and Prewriting

Toni was a 5-year-old with a seizure disorder and an anxiety disorder. She was very interactive socially and verbally but resisted all fine motor and paper-and-pencil activities. The occupational therapy evaluation indicated difficulty with accuracy in reach, grasp, and release because of deficits in visual perception and motor control. Toni's favorite activity was eating. She often talked about her favorite foods and loved to pretend she was eating. Her family wanted Toni to participate in academic-oriented paper-and-pencil activities. Because of Toni's resistance to using a pencil, the occupational therapist determined it was best to start with embedding the visual constructional aspects of prewriting first. She decided to use craft sticks to have Toni imitate making intersecting lines for a cross. When presented with the craft sticks activity, Toni turned and walked away, refusing to come back.

The occupational therapist planned a playful approach for the next session. The occupational therapist decided to capitalize on the fact that craft sticks are quite similar to sticks used in food items. In the next session, the occupational therapist first held the sticks, pretended to lick one, and began banging the sticks on the table as she sang "Lollipop, lollipop, ohhh, lolli-, lolli-pop." Toni smiled and watched the therapist, laughing as the therapist added an exclamatory "pop!" as she put her sticks together to make a cross and put them on the table in crossed position. Toni asked to play too, and they sang several rounds with Toni actively trying to place the craft sticks in a cross formation.

Learning Activity

Considering the case of Toni, how could you address the work of prewriting differently using play?

---

also need to come up with unique approaches for children who find prewriting more work than play. For example, making intersecting lines for a railroad crossing sign may not be work for a child who is very interested in trains. But even using a pencil may be resisted by some children, and more creative playful approaches are needed such as presented in the Handwriting Without Tears pre-K readiness activities and illustrated in the case of Toni.

Unique ways of drawing can also be more playful. For example, faces can be drawn with washable markers and squirted with water to "melt" them, or they can be drawn on partially inflated balloons and then blown to "stretch the monster face" or "make a silly face."

Infusing Play into Cutting

Cutting with scissors is another common referral concern for pediatric occupational therapists. Typically, the child has unusual challenges in developing this skill and thus perceives it as more work than play. This contrasts with the reaction of typical children who may show great pride in their developing cutting skills. For the child who is uninterested in or resistive to using scissors, the following suggestions may help in transforming cutting into a playful activity:

- Use scissors as puppet mouths to "talk" to each other
- Use scissors as mouths to "eat" paper
- Snip small pieces of paper as cargo to load a truck/ train, as food for a character, or as raindrops to fall
- Make a path on paper with stamps/stickers of monsters or dinosaurs and then "chase"/"eat" them with the scissors
- Place a sticker at the beginning and end of the line, such as a dog at the beginning and a bone at the end, or a car at one end and a house at the other, etc.
- Cut different materials, such as play-dough and straws
- Cut a small amount at the end of each pass through an obstacle course or scooter board path
- Cut items that can be used as props in play:
  - Costumes out of paper and tape—color, cut, and tape things onto clothes (clowns with red circles, spots on a dog, red nose for "Rudolph")
  - Trace, color, and cut large numbers to make a sports jersey
  - Cut items to make paper dolls, dogs, super heroes, etc.

Minimizing the Work in "Play" Activities

Even activities that are commonly called play and seen as play by other children in the general society may not be experienced as play by individual pediatric clients. For example, some children are not interested in any of the play that the other children are doing at recess or in their neighborhoods. Thus, the children play by themselves. This is problematic when the child wants to have friends or needs to develop social interaction skills. One possible solution is offering other play activities (such as board games at recess) or getting other children to play what the client wants to play. Another option is building skills so that the child can join successfully in the activities the children are playing. But often these two approaches are inadequate. The reality is that the other children may not share the client's interest or may lack in-depth knowledge to play games based on the client's interest (such as detailed knowledge about how solar systems are created, or all the countries and capitals of the world). Furthermore, even with foundational skills, some children will not be motivated to play what other children are playing. In such cases, recasting the game into play for a particular client is needed. If the client can perceive it as play, he or she will be more motivated to participate in the activity. The gap between the interests of a client and the play context can be bridged with knowledge of activity analysis and evaluation of the child, as in the case of Zach.

Extending Limited Play Interests

Some children have very limited interests. For some children, their interests are so limited that they do not display any self-initiated attempts to engage in activities. They may not be interested in the objects available, and they may show no interest in other children's play. They may not have the skills to engage, or they may not have had a positive experience with an activity. They may not object to the therapist's ideas, but it can be very difficult to find activities in which they genuinely enjoy participating. For other children, their interests are so strong and compelling that they are very resistive to anything outside of those interests. In these situations, the occupational therapist is challenged to help pediatric clients extend their interests in order to participate in and experience play in a diversity of activities, places, and social settings.

Lack of Interest. At times, it can be hard to find anything that interests a child. In these cases, the occupational therapist must create occupational appeal (Munier, Myers, & Pierce, 2008) and focus on the precursors of play (Holloway, 2008). Again, this process starts with the occupational therapy evaluation, where even limited interests are identified to support active engagement by the child. For example, a child may like a particular character,

---

Zach and Recess

Zach was a 9-year-old attending a full-inclusion classroom. He liked other people and had a strong desire for social interaction with all ages of children and adults. At recess, however, he mostly played by himself, enacting elaborate make-believe stories of kind animals that play together and avoid attacks by "mean" animals. The other children played soccer during recess. When asked if he wanted to play with the other children, Zach responded "yes" but said that he did not want to play soccer because "it is mean and you get hurt." Although some other activities were available, the other children still wanted to play soccer. If Zach was going to play with the other children, he would need to be able to play soccer, and he would need to be willing to play soccer. The occupational therapist decided to combine Zach's interest in a make-believe story with soccer. Together in their sessions, they made up a story book about horses and wolves playing "soccer" (see **Appendix 7–2**). Then, Zach was willing to try playing soccer.

Learning Activity

Considering the case of Zach, how could you address the work of recess differently using play?

---

or something as simple as the color red or shiny objects. These materials can be used in therapy as objects toward which the child will move or reach. Or the child may show a strength with visual perception and thus be more inclined to find constructional activities intrinsically satisfying. This is the opening for the occupational therapist to "get into" the play of a child with limited interests.

The occupational therapist does not stop here. Extending such a narrow interest into broader engagement in daily activities requires a continually graded approach. As the child consistently shows interest in actively participating, the occupational therapist upgrades the challenge so that there is a delay in reaching/obtaining the object, or more complex ways of using the object. For example, if the child likes shiny red objects, the occupational therapist may place shiny red beads easily within a child's reach and gradually move some farther away to sustain engagement while working on trunk rotation. The occupational therapist may place an object of interest in a tunnel, at the top of a structure, or behind another object

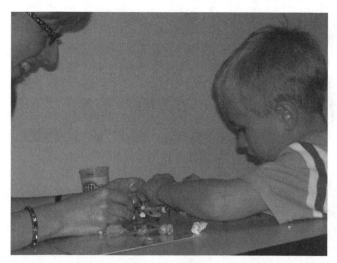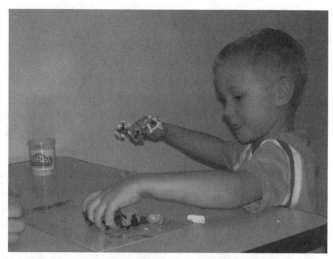

An occupational therapist demonstrates respect for, and valuing of, a child's play interests in toy vehicles by incorporating these toys in a fine motor play activity of rolling small play-dough snow balls to cover a plane's propellers in a pretend blizzard.

to encourage a child to crawl, climb, or negotiate obstacles. To promote play, the occupational therapist grades the challenge so that the child is continually able to *obtain* the object of interest and experience the pleasure of doing so. Momentum is created that encourages further repetition and perseverance with the occupation (Carlson, 1996). Once the child is willing to participate in a broader range of activities, the occupational therapist can create greater opportunities for practice and skill development. As occupational therapists balance out the child's limited interests and the goals desired for the child's future, they reflect on this question: Is this a step that helps the child move forward in making therapeutic gains toward his or her goals? If the answer is in the affirmative, therapists can know that their reasoning is sound.

Narrow Interests and Opposition. Some children get so focused on their own particular interests or ways of doing things that anything else is met with great opposition and resistance. The client reacts as if all the therapist's ideas are work. The therapist must self-reflect on his or her own interactions with the child to verify that one's therapeutic use of self is playful for that individual child. Additional careful analysis of activities is done, and the occupational therapist plans creative activities that are both playful and therapeutic so that clients will try to actively participate, as the case of Javier illustrates.

Some children are extremely resistant to adult direction. The gap between what the child wants to do and what the child needs to do is big. In some cases, the occupational therapist will opt to give the client choices or turns in selecting activities. But sometimes, even this step

is too big initially. In such cases, the occupational therapist starts where the child is and builds a bridge through a series of very carefully graded activities. Each activity modification is a small step toward the goal, as the case of Paul illustrates.

An older child can be involved directly in the explicit process of combining elements of what he or she wants and needs to do. Clients can be informed that a particular area needs to be addressed and why (e.g., "balance needs to be improved to play on the playground without getting hurt"), and the therapist then gathers the child's ideas for how to do this. For other children, it can be framed as a social interaction dilemma of needing to find a way for both ideas to be included and played together. For example, to explicate this process and make it seem fair, both therapist and child can write their top ideas for the session on different index cards and then pair index cards from each one into a single activity. In one case, one client came up with an idea of playing space travel (on his index card) to visit aliens and return to earth, and then writing (on the therapist's index card) a letter to the aliens about the visit to thank them for the interesting food and so on. In another case, when a child saw the cards of his choices, he stated, "Wow, I can't wait! There is so much fun stuff to do!"

Limited Interests and Social Play. Extending limited play interests can be especially important for enhancing social play. Many children who have limited play interests have an interest different from that of their potential playmates. If a client is not interested in playing what the other children are playing, and the other children lack the knowledge or interest to play what the client is playing, socially

Javier, Interests, and Resistance

Javier was a 7-year-old with obsessive compulsive disorder and ADHD. He was being seen for poor motor planning and postural control because his parents wanted him to be able to imitate others' movements in play and various after-school activities and to be able to move safely around the environment (without bumping into stable objects). Javier was not very interested in anything in the clinic. He loved to talk perseveratively about his various interests or things that were on his mind. When he talked, he was unable to initiate or continue a therapeutic activity because he had to stop to talk. Thus, his talking about his interests was a barrier to engagement in therapeutic activities. It was very difficult to interrupt or stop this narrative.

One of Javier's interests became the *Miss Nelson* book series (Allard, 1985, 1988). He liked to pretend to transform into the character Coach Swamp and have the therapist "athlete" do "exercises" (run around). Although this activity helped build rapport between the occupational therapist and Javier, she wanted to adapt this activity to provide additional therapeutic gains and increase variety in play. Because "exercises" could be therapeutic, the occupational therapist decided to develop "Coach Swamp" exercises. She made cards with pictures and labels of different exercises that would help Javier build kinesthetic awareness and postural control. She presented these "Coach Swamp" exercise cards to Javier, telling him he could pick which ones to do. As the therapist played the role of the lazy student athlete, she explained how she did not know how to do each exercise and would need the coach to show and teach her. Thus, "coach" Javier demonstrated each exercise and did them alongside the occupational therapist "athlete." The exercises were transformed from work into a specific preferred play activity as Javier adjusted to novelty in his play.

Learning Activity

Considering the case of Javier, how else could you address his narrow interests and resistance therapeutically in play?

Tommy, Interests, and Social Play

Tommy was a bright and smiling 7-year-old who loved maps. He had a library of atlases at home and was particularly fond of Antarctica and any stories of the explorers who traveled with Sir Ernest Shackleton. Tommy's peers were less than interested in this topic, and Tommy generally had few friends to play with at recess. His occupational therapist was able to create a game for Tommy that allowed him to engage with his peers in a way that was fun and developmentally appropriate for them but that also engaged him in an area in which he was quite interested. The occupational therapist created a "tag"-like game that provided rough and tumble play and recreated the adventures of Shackleton in the exploration of the arctic. The occupational therapist set the situation so that the boys each got to add a rule to the game; and Tommy got to tell the boys if the rule matched the real story of the adventure (so he got to share his knowledge), and the boys got to make up a fun game with the rules they wanted for the game. The game included some sharing and working together (the explorers had to work together to survive), some rough and tumble climbing and racing (who could make it to the top of the mountain first), and lots of sensory motor activity on the playground (pulling, pushing, hauling) as the boys acted out the explorer's adventures.

Learning Activity

Considering the case of Tommy, how else could you address his limited interests to extend his participation in social play?

interactive play that is truly playful does not occur. Extending this limited play interest in ways that encompass what other children can and will want to play creates opportunities for social play to emerge. Elements of both play preferences can be fused together to create a new activity, such as combining ponies and *Star Wars* characters to make up a new story that two different children can play together. Tag games are social games that have been successfully modified to accomodate a child's unique interest (Baker, Koegel, & Koegel, 1998), as described in the case of Tommy.

Individuals with disabilities can feel that their different strengths and interests are devalued and unimportant if the focus is just on others' conventional interests. At the same time, only engaging in their own unique interests without regard for others limits their ability to interact with and negotiate the social world. Including the interests of both the child and others shows that both are valued and respected.

■ PREPARING FOR THE UNPREDICTABLE: ADAPTING ACTIVITIES IN THE MOMENT TO PROMOTE PLAY

As noted in Chapter Six, therapy is a dynamic process that requires the occupational therapist's ongoing assessment, analysis, and adaptation on a moment-by-moment basis, especially when focused on play. Although the treatment plan is a guide for therapy, a variety of unanticipated events will occur in each treatment session. The occupational therapist cannot predict the child's exact response to an activity or the opportunities that may emerge. The child may like or dislike all aspects or some part of the activity. The child may be having a challenging day and may be tired, frustrated, or agitated. The child may be having a very positive day and may be very agreeable and more playful than usual. The occupational therapist has to be attentive to both challenges and possibilities that emerge and be flexible to adapt to these changes. The occupational therapist stays flexible to recognize and understand changes in the child's emotional state, needs, and desires. Adjusting in the moment takes fast thinking and thus requires that the therapist be prepared; he or she must complete activity analyses beforehand—maintain a clear picture of the child's overall strengths, needs, and goals; and have a sound knowledge of play. The actual methods for achieving therapy goals must be changeable on a moment-by-moment basis to match where the child is at that moment.

Recognizing and Extending Opportunities for Play

By having a clear vision of what play is and focusing on the child's overall goals rather than a specific planned activity, the occupational therapist is poised to adapt activities during the session to be playlike. Hints of play may occur briefly and unexpectedly, and the occupational therapist must be ready to seize these opportunities. It may be a comment, a sound, or a movement (Spitzer, 2008). It may be the first time the child does something new or more complicated (even if by chance). The child may merely glance at a person or object, or even suggest an idea. The occupational therapist, then, can scaffold the child's play by providing just enough guidance or assistance for the child to initiate or continue a play activity (Baranek, Reinhartsen, & Wannamaker, 2001), as illustrated in the case of Allison.

To promote play and the child's intrinsic drive, the occupational therapist avoids stopping the child or saying no to his or her ideas. Instead, the occupational therapist immediately thinks of *how* to do what the child wants to do, and how to adapt the activity to make it happen. Certainly, because of potential safety hazards, institutional policies, or physical circumstances, the occupational therapist sometimes must place some limits on the child's ideas. Even with safety concerns that limit play in the moment, the occupational therapist still searches for alternative ways to let the child play. For example, Daniel was a child with Asperger's syndrome who always wanted to do stunts, such as flying flips from the trapeze, for which the therapist could not ensure his safety. Therefore, his occupational therapist consulted with Daniel's mother to encourage a gymnastics class focused on trapeze acts. Daniel became a very good trapeze artist and looked forward to these special opportunities for physically extreme play. If play is the goal, to the greatest extent possible, the occupational therapist places the child's input foremost and then thinks of *how* to make it happen, as illustrated in the case of Thomas.

In-the-moment, ongoing clinical reasoning is necessary because an occupational therapist cannot know everything, past and evolving, that is happening in a client's life. Therefore, the therapist must be open to new information, skills, and interests that provide new options for intervention and play.

Paul, Interests, and Opposition

Paul was a 3-year-old with autism. His parents had great difficulty finding providers who would work with him because of his extreme anger with any adult attempts at intervention. His tantrums were frequent and extreme in volume, aggression, and duration. Even when someone tried to help him do what he wanted, he would throw a tantrum. His language was severely limited. Even with explanations and demonstrations, he did not seem to understand that the adult was trying to help him. The occupational therapy evaluation found restricted play interests. He preferred rough physical play and novel nontoy items (such as a flashlight, pencil sharpener, etc.), and he liked to watch cartoons; hold, throw, and mouth balls; roll cars on different surfaces; and dump, kick, throw, or step on most other toys. He appreciated positive emotional reactions from adults such as smiling with praise, "yeah's," and clapping. His gross motor skills were well developed for his age, and he seemed to rely on visual learning. Given the nature of his interests, he could be very destructive and had to be monitored closely and continuously by adults.

Because any involvement in what Paul was doing would be met with tantrums, the occupational therapist opted to let Paul engage in what he selected, monitor him for safety, and model play with selected other materials in strategic locations so that he would notice her. The occupational therapist selected one item at a time that she believed Paul was likely to enjoy based on his other interests and with which she believed he would be successful. For example, she selected a number of sensory-motor materials that gave sensory feedback. Given his visual strengths, she also determined that constructional play would be a likely category of play that Paul could perform. Therefore, she used blocks that she stacked up and then knocked down. She used long blocks laid out like a road with a car to drive on the "road"; she gradually offered other constructional activities as well.

With the occupational therapist's modeling of play, Paul began to come over and imitate what she had done. He began indicating that he wanted the occupational therapist to get an item for him, which gave the occupational therapist another dimension to her role in his expanding play repertoire. Gradually, over the course of these first 2 months, she had established a small role in his play. Initially, he took over each activity and would not allow the occupational therapist to be involved. Then, over the course of the next 4 months, the occupational therapist began to establish "turns," first in parallel by repeating the activity Paul had done with extra materials and emphasizing "my turn" and "your turn" with gestures. Later, the occupational therapist was able to bring out a construction/demolition game, "Don't Break the Ice." She very quickly took her turn between each of his turns at hitting the blocks. Eventually, she was able to get Paul to wait for her to take a turn. In this way, Paul was learning to tolerate adult interaction, laying the groundwork for further intervention, and he was broadening his play repertoire to participate in social play and play with constructional toys in a safe and independent manner.

Allison and a New Play Opportunity

Allison was a preschooler with autism and limited language. One of her occupational therapy goals was to initiate (select) play activities. She was just beginning to initiate activities and spontaneous language appropriately. Her speech-language therapist recommended that adults try to respond contingently to her language because she often said words that seemed to lack meaning in the current situation. By responding accurately to the words, it was reasoned, Allison would begin to understand the meaning of the words.

During this session, Allison had selected a swing. Her occupational therapist was asking her what she wanted to throw. The therapist and Allison's mother were giving ideas when suddenly Allison said, "triangle." There was no obvious triangle visible in the room, and this seemed like a random, possibly meaningless word. Thus, Allison's mother explained, "You can't throw a triangle. There's no triangle." Although Allison's mother was correct, the occupational therapist wanted to seize on Allison's rare initiation and offered, "If you want a triangle, you can throw *to* a triangle." She quickly cut a triangle out of colored construction paper and taped it to the floor for Allison to throw bean bags to it. Whether Allison's comment was an intentional idea for the activity is unclear, but her occupational therapist's valuing and integrating Allison's input are clear.

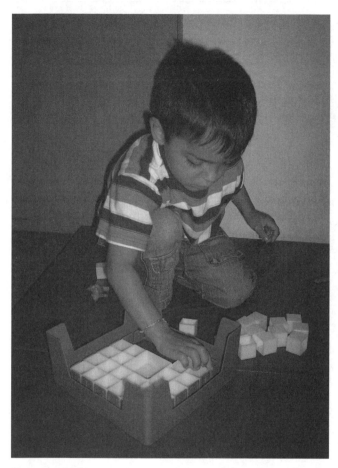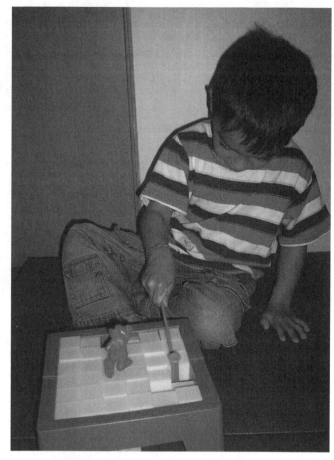

Strengths and interest in construction and destruction play themes may be blended with a cooperative turn-taking game to build tolerance for social play with a game of "Don't Break the Ice."

Thomas and an Unexpected Play Opportunity

Thomas was a bright first grader with autism. He loved school work and preferred to do workbooks and read in his leisure time. He was receiving occupational therapy to increase his play skills, praxis, and postural control to engage in a variety of leisure activities, especially with other children. He preferred play themes related to categories of knowledge and information such as animals from different parts of the world. He was not interested in pretend games of being the animals or in various topics in which his classmates were interested. He always read books at the beginning and end of each session in the waiting room. He often asked the therapist to read a book to him. She usually redirected him through such comments as "it is time to play." Reading was not a goal of therapy and seemed to be a detractor from therapy.

On one day when Thomas was a little more insistent, asking to take the book into the therapy room, his occupational therapist agreed to the request as long as he stood on a balance cushion to read it; and he agreed. When he finished, he put the book down and told her that he had another book to read, and before she could respond, he immediately held his hands together like a book and began a long stream of memorized words about a Spider-Man story. As soon as he paused, the occupational therapist offered "Let's play Spider-Man!" "Okay," said Thomas. The occupational therapist stated that Thomas would *be* Spider-Man and began asking Thomas who the "bad guy, villains" were. Thomas gave her some names. They set up targets to be these named villains, and Thomas threw bean bag "spider-webs" at them with excitement at getting the bad guys. Thomas had accepted the Spider-Man role and expanded his play because his occupational therapist was flexible and adapted to Thomas' needs and desires in the moment.

Learning Activity

View the video clips of the occupational therapy sessions (you will be reviewing the same clips you reviewed for the therapeutic use of self learning activity in Chapter Four).

This time, as you view these videos, complete the Video Review Form in **Appendix 7-3** (also available online at *www.jbpub.com*) to help you increase your understanding of creating and adapting play in pediatric occupational therapy.

■ CONCLUSION

Incorporating play in pediatric occupational therapy is clearly both occupation-focused, and client-centered. Various of ways to incorporate play were detailed in this chapter. Although the child referred to occupational therapy often experiences a range of daily activities as work, through occupational therapy, they can be transformed into play or playlike experiences. Based on activity analysis and the child's input, the occupational therapist can plan therapeutic activities that are also play. The spontaneous and dynamic aspects of play are difficult to plan with certainty. However, with a strong foundation in activity analysis, knowledge of play, and awareness of the child's interests, the occupational therapist is well positioned for this formidable and rewarding aspect of practice and is ready to seize spontaneous opportunities to create play in the moment.

Appendix 7-1

Pediatric Occupational Therapy Treatment Plan

Pediatric Occupational Therapy Treatment Plan

Child's Name: _____   Date of Birth: _____

Diagnosis: _____

Developed by: _____ , Occupational Therapist

Signature _____   Date: _____

Child's Interests:

Hand Dominance: Right   Left   Other: _____

Precautions: _____

Child Strengths and Concerns (as of _____)	Goals (set on _____)	Treatment Approach (Activities and Adaptations)

Comments/Note(s):

Appendix 7-2

Example of Zach's Story from Occupational Therapy

Horses vs. Wolves

The horses lived on one side of the forest and wolves lived on the other side.

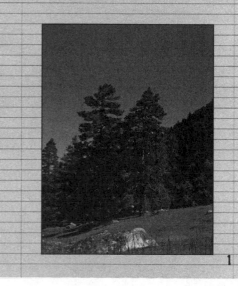

1

One day, they woke up. The horses tried to kick a big rock to knock down the wolves' den made out of rocks. The wolves tried to kick the big rock to knock down the horses' house made of wood. Sometimes, the wolves hit the horses' house and sometimes the horses hit the wolves' den. Each time, it hurt their home and they tried to get even with the other side. Sometimes, the wolves blocked the horses' rock and kicked it back at their house. Sometimes, the horses blocked the wolves' rock and kicked it back at their den.

2

Sometimes a horse or wolf got hit by the rock. They didn't get hurt. They just got a little dizzy and they got up and kept kicking.

3

Sometimes one horse was blocked by the wolves so it kicked the rock to another horse who could kick it at the wolves' den. Sometimes one wolf was blocked by the horses so it kicked the rock to another wolf who could kick it at the horses' house.

4

They kept kicking and kicking until the afternoon. The moon started coming up and they got tired. They dropped the rock and fell on the ground and went to sleep. zzzzzzzzzzzzzzzzzzz

5

The next morning they got up and started kicking again.

6

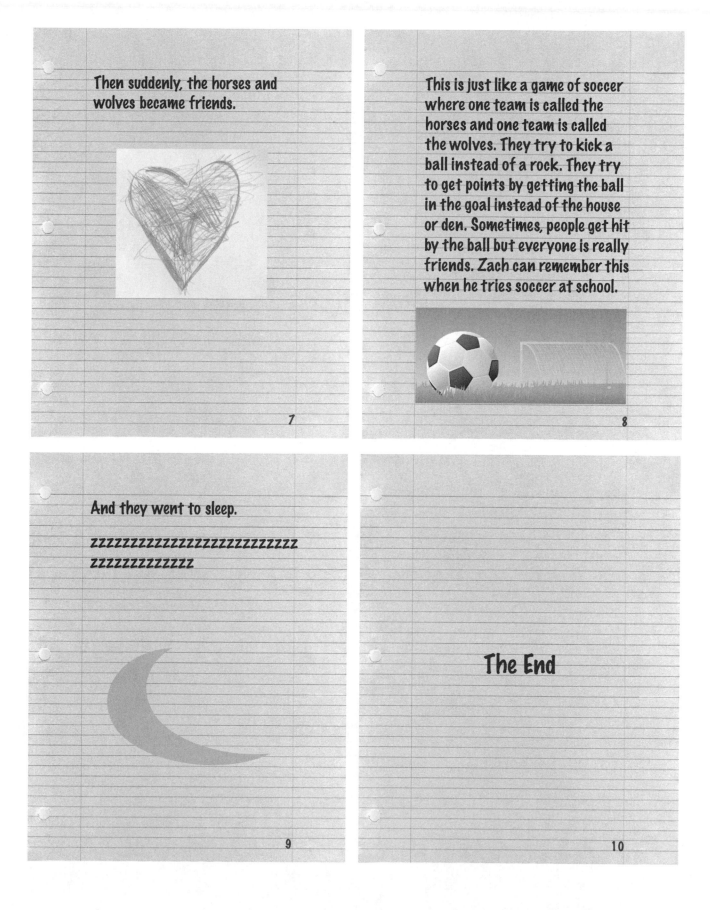

Then suddenly, the horses and wolves became friends.

7

This is just like a game of soccer where one team is called the horses and one team is called the wolves. They try to kick a ball instead of a rock. They try to get points by getting the ball in the goal instead of the house or den. Sometimes, people get hit by the ball but everyone is really friends. Zach can remember this when he tries soccer at school.

8

And they went to sleep.

ZZZZZZZZZZZZZZZZZZZZZZZZZZ
ZZZZZZZZZZZZ

9

The End

10

Appendix 7-3

Video Review Form for Creating Play in Pediatric Occupational Therapy Sessions

Video Review Form for Creating Play

Directions: Use this form to guide your viewing of each video treatment session to increase your understanding of selecting, creating, and adapting play in pediatric occupational therapy.

How did the activity relate to the child's interests?

How did the activity relate to the child's needs?

How was each treatment activity graded (positioning, resistance, duration/endurance, distance/ mobility, coordination/dexterity, sensory perceptual characteristics, cognition, developmental level, social interaction)?

How was the therapeutic work play-like?

What adaptations did the therapist have to make in the moment of therapy?

8

Creative Play Applications in Specific Aspects of Pediatric Practice

After reading this chapter the reader will

1. Discuss clinical reasoning and strategies to balance flexibility with structure to promote play.

2. List strategies in grading pretend play, challenge, competition, and fear and danger themes in play.

3. Describe the value of including super hero play in pediatric occupational therapy.

4. Explain challenges and considerations for occupational therapists when presented with family play, adolescent play, and problematic or underground play themes.

5. Discuss considerations with incorporating challenge, setting limits on play, and integrating obsessive play themes.

> *The creation of something new is not accomplished by the intellect but by the play instinct.*
> —Carl Jung

A number of particular dilemmas commonly arise with using play in pediatric occupational therapy. Given their frequency and complexity, these dilemmas merit individual review in this chapter. For each practice dilemma, the approach is the same as advocated in previous chapters—creatively adapting activities to be an attainable challenge, to be enjoyable, and to be what the child wants to do. This is not a comprehensive listing of problems and solutions because we cannot anticipate all the challenges posed by the variety of clients with and contexts in which occupational therapists work. Therefore, the specifics in this chapter are designed to provide examples of how to plan for and adjust therapy plans to contend with the real challenges of therapy in particular situations. These examples address structure, pretend play, challenge and competition, danger and fear themes, underground play, family play, excessive play, obsessive play, and adolescent play. Given multiple exemplars, you will be better able to adapt to other challenges as well.

■ ADAPTING STRUCTURE IN PLAY TO BALANCE FLEXIBILITY

Sometimes novelty and spontaneity must be graded for what the child can tolerate. In wanting to encourage play, pediatric occupational therapists try to share as much control as possible with the child, allowing for flexibility and novelty to encourage the spontaneity that characterizes real play. Nonetheless, some children prefer high levels of structure and routine and have trouble tolerating the uncertainty of novelty and flexibility, or they get very disorganized in unstructured environments. To encourage play and internal organization, the occupational therapist generally tries to limit externally imposed structure and organization as much as possible. Balancing between structure and flexibility involves ongoing clinical reasoning based on sound activity analysis to increase the child's enjoyment and to grade the "just right" challenge. Providing choices and developing routines are two strategies for adapting flexibility and structure in play (**Table 8-1**).

Providing Choices

Occupational therapists desire to give children as much choice as possible to include their interests. This involves getting the child's input. However, some children cannot

Table 8-1   Strategies for Adapting Flexibility and Structure in Play

Providing choices

- Ask the child which activity or material he or she wants to use (grading the range available from which to select).
- Show two or more items.
- Show pictures of two or more items.
- Offer an activity consistent with child's movements (e.g., jumping), eye gaze, sounds, etc.

Developing routines

- Use a similar structure/organization (sequence of steps, materials, time, etc.).
- Provide an explicit schedule (see **Figure 8-1**).
- Use visual supports (pictures or words).
- Give reminders about upcoming transitions.
- Use key phrases and gestures to indicate and reinforce the order (e.g., first, next, last).
- Develop rules for an activity.

make a choice, show initiation toward an activity, or identify potential choices. In such cases, the therapist may suggest something that is similar to the movement the child is doing. For example, if the child is jumping around, the occupational therapist might suggest a structured jumping game, such as jumping from one spot to another, jumping over something, or jumping on a trampoline. The therapist may show the child two toys or two pictures of activities and see which one the child selects, reaches/leans toward, or gazes at (Van Tubbergen, Warschausky, Birnholz, & Baker, 2008).

Providing choices must also be adapted for the individual child's needs, abilities, and therapeutic goals. The number and type of items offered or the field from which to select should be graded to provide structure. For example, some children may be overwhelmed by a large number of options. This child may need to start with a limited number and then gradually tolerate increased options. A child with ideation problems may have difficulty identifying anything to do during unstructured play time and may require different adaptations, such as suggestions of "let's pick something your friends are doing [at recess]" or "let's see what games there are [on the playground]."

Developing Routines

Many children find reassurance in a basic routine so they know what to expect next. Some clients have trouble understanding a general implicit flow of a therapy session, and the uncertainty can cause emotional distress or disorganization. For example, some children may repeatedly ask about what is next, when will _____ happen, will they be doing _____ today. Others may act out with a transition to another activity because it was unexpected, or they thought they were going to follow the same series of activities as last time. In such situations, the occupational therapist must make the implicit flow more explicit and structured to help the child participate. Grading structure is important to balance with the need for flexibility. Children who thrive on structure can easily become dependent on the structure and lose out on opportunities for spontaneous play because it is "not time" for a spontaneous play activity. The more open the routine is, the more the therapist can take advantage of opportunities or new information that may arise within a treatment session. The occupational therapist provides just enough graded structure to help the child participate as illustrated by the case of Christopher (Baron, 1991; Moor, 2002).

The amount and type of structure are graded to match the child's needs and therapeutic goals. Some children need a general routine or structure for a session and daily activities, and others need a detailed, structured schedule (see Figure 8-1 for examples in therapy sessions). A general category or time may be enough, or exact details may be needed. For example, it may be enough to list "get dressed," or it may be necessary to list all the steps to getting dressed. Many children simply need to know what they are transitioning toward in order to end the activity they are doing. Visual supports (pictures or written words) may be necessary for a child who has difficulty with language processing. Reminders throughout the session may also be needed to help the child prepare for transitions.

Individual activities can easily be structured by establishing time limits or other end points or making an activity into a game with rules. Several websites have freely available games and game board templates that can be downloaded and customized for a particular child's needs.[1]

■ ADAPTING FROM CONCRETE TO PRETEND PLAY

Although imaginative play can be a very powerful way to engage children in therapeutic activities (Parham, 1992),

---

[1] *http://jc-schools.net/tutorials/gameboard.htm*
http://www.activityvillage.co.uk/kids_games_and_activities.htm
http://www.speakingofspeech.com/Therapy_Games.html

Christopher and Structure

Christopher was a 4-year-old with cerebral palsy and an anxiety disorder. Because his occupational therapist was committed to promoting play and his intrinsic motivation, she consistently asked Christopher what he wanted to do. In the first few sessions, he was unable to offer any ideas, so the occupational therapist suggested some activities. Then Christopher began telling the therapist what he wanted to do (an activity from a previous session). Eventually, he wanted to do the same series of activities in the same order. Christopher's occupational therapist wanted to encourage more variation in play and skills, so she began to suggest different activities or changes in the activity. Each time he screamed and cried "no" and said the activity he wanted. At this point, it became very difficult to get him to calm and try the alternate activity. The occupational therapist recognized that this level of change and flexibility was too disorganizing for Christopher. At the same time, the occupational therapist also recognized that with this inflexible preference for predictable structure, Christopher could become dependent on a rigid structure. Therefore, the occupational therapist introduced a simple structure of alternating between the child's choice and the occupational therapist's choice for an activity, and Christopher's tantrums subsided. Initially, she provided warnings and reminders about these changes with emotional assurances that this would be fun. She sometimes used Christopher's ideas during her choice times. Eventually, with preparing Christopher, she also alternated whose choice was first each session and the number of choices per session.

Figure 8-1   Examples of Variation in Structured Routines for Pediatric Occupational Therapy Sessions

Example 1	Example 2
My choice/turn	Body/gym activities
Your choice/turn	Snack
My choice/turn	Get my things
Your choice/turn	Go home/Go to class

Example 3	Example 4
Use ball	Take shoes off
Play game at table	Swing
Write	Write
Walk to class	Obstacle Course
	Craft
	Put shoes on
	Wait for mommy and _____ to talk
	Walk to car
	Drive to park

some children need help to participate in pretend play. Even when they have the foundational cognitive skills of at least 18 months developmentally (Stagnitti & Unsworth, 2000), pretend play can still be difficult. This is very common in children with autism (Moor, 2002), who tend to do better with concrete rather than abstract thinking. When you suggest pretending, the child may tell you, "I'm not Superman, I'm Peter" or "That's not a phone, it's a block." In such cases, the occupational therapist may have to grade activities carefully, slowly introducing pretend components into the child's current play. This can be done in several ways (**Table 8-2**).

It is often best to start pretend play with objects related to the child's own body and behavior because this tends to occur first in typical development (Hellendoorn,

1994). The development of pretend play and related age expectations as described in Chapter One can provide a basis for this process. For example, as described, functional or presymbolic play involves the use of real or real-looking objects or props in conventional ways. Pretending to drink from a cup, eat from a spoon, sleep with a pillow, and talk on a "phone" are examples of the most basic form of pretending. Because the "pretending" is very concrete and closely related to the real use of objects, it can be easier for a child to understand and enjoy doing (Moor, 2002). Gradually expanding the type of objects and the way they are used allows the child to gain foundational pretend play skills. For example, real objects can also be used in relation to someone else (such as pretending to feed a parent or sibling) or to a doll or other toy character. Expanding symbolic play next involves the use of "real" props such as a fireman's hat, pretend dishes, or pretend lawnmower. Then the occupational therapist may introduce using objects that merely resemble a real object. For example, a plastic banana may be a "phone," a rectangular block may be a "candy bar," a red ball may be a "strawberry," and so on. The more closely the object resembles the true item in size, color, and shape, the more easily it may be accepted by the

Table 8-2   Strategies for Adapting Concrete Play to Pretend Play

- Grade development from concrete to pretend play by using:
  - Real objects and actions related to child's body (e.g., pretend to drink from a cup)
  - Real objects and actions related to another body (e.g., parent) or doll/toy
  - Realistic props (e.g., firefighter's hat)
  - Alternative objects with a resemblance to the real represented object (e.g., rectangular block as a "candy bar")
  - Alternative objects without a clear resemblance to the real represented object (e.g., a purple ball as a "candy bar")
  - Absence of real object (completely imagined object)
  - A role:
    - Reality-based role (e.g., mother, police officer, doctor)
    - Fantasy roles (e.g., super hero, horse)
  - Narrative plots
    - A familiar plot from a favorite book or video
    - Novel plots or combining plots from two or more stories (e.g., Superman and Star Wars)
- Model pretend play
- Emphasize difference between "pretend" and "real"
- Explore how an object or action is "like" something else
- Use favorite interests
- Use a prop to signify changes in role from "real" to "pretend"
- Develop a story to explain the pretend play activity

child. A small red ball looks more like a strawberry than a big purple ball does, but eventually even a big purple ball may become a strawberry during pretend play.

As with most play skills, the occupational therapist will have to balance the opportunity to repeat, practice, and master each new pretend play skill with encouraging further expansion of these themes. As pretend play is learned, each child will need different amounts of time to practice this new skill by repeating the pretend play. Just like learning to use stairs, some children will want to repeat the same pretend sequence extensively before they are ready to expand it. As these are repeated, the occupational therapist may grade the introduction of other pretend play into these repetitions.

The occupational therapist may initially emphasize use of the words "pretend" and "not real" to help the child understand and accept the imaginative play ideas: "We are doing *pretend* eating, *not real* eating." The child may need to observe first before feeling comfortable to try pretend play. The occupational therapist can model these strategies by applying them to him- or herself.

Many children enjoy pretending favorite story lines from books or films because they already know the story well and do not have to come up with unique pretend ideas. A child may be more open to recreating in pretend play other areas of real interest as well, as in the case of Olivia. In this way, the occupational therapist helps the child connect pretend play to the child's interests and dreams. Pretend play becomes more than just a skill, but a truly enjoyable occupation.

At older developmental levels, the occupational therapist may want to encourage themes and narrative plots because this tends to become the more dominant form of pretend play. Usually, this involves the child becoming someone else, such as a super hero, pirate, firefighter, ballerina, Olympic star, mother, pilot, or animal. Pretending to be someone else

---

Olivia and Pretend Play

Olivia loved board games but resisted pretend play. Whenever the occupational therapist suggested a pretend theme, Olivia asked the therapist questions such as what was she doing and why was she doing it. Despite encouragement, modeling, and explanations, Olivia would comply with a direction to do a particular action but never initiated or responded spontaneously to various pretend play themes. Instead, Olivia repeatedly asked to play her current favorite games of Perfection and Mouse Trap. To combine Olivia's interests in board games with therapeutic goals to increase variation and flexibility in play, the occupational therapist suggested that they create large pretend versions of the games in the form of obstacle courses. Olivia was delighted with this idea and actively participated with designing and going through the game "boards" as she actively pretended to be the game "pieces." From this base, as the occupational therapist explained how other pretend themes were similar to pretending Perfection and Mouse Trap, Olivia happily accepted more pretend play themes offered by her therapist and then other children.

can present a significant difficulty for some children who resist this notion. It can be helpful to start with "real people" roles, such as a firefighter or mother, because the child has seen these roles and knows that people really can be mothers or firefighters. Pretending to ride a horse is closer to real life than pretending to be a horse. Other children may be more receptive to characters and story lines with which they are familiar in favorite books, movies, and television shows. Later, the child may become more open to pretending something unreal, such as a unicorn or Superman.

To start, the occupational therapist may simply comment on how what the child is doing is "like" something else; for example, "you are flying through the air (on a swing) like birds fly in the air." The occupational therapist may need to clarify, "you are *not* a bird, but you are doing what birds do, so you are *like* a bird, you are a *pretend* bird." The occupational therapist may even encourage the child to think of other things that are "like" this, for example, other things that fly. Again, emphasizing the use of the words "pretend" and "not real" can help the child understand and accept the imaginative play ideas. The occupational therapist may also model pretend play so that the child can observe this phenomenon before asking the child to think of him- or herself differently. A prop that signifies the role change, such as a firefighter hat or cape, may also help the child to differentiate or mark between the world of make-believe and the everyday real world. A story written to explain the concepts that can be read multiple times may also help the child to understand and develop internal control over this form of play. (See **Appendix 8-1** for sources to assist in writing therapeutic stories.) The *Miss Nelson* book series (Allard, 1985, 1988) is an example of a story of how a person can pretend to be different people.

■ SUPER HERO PLAY AND SELF-EFFICACY

As described in Chapter One, playing a super hero is a common form of pretend play for children (Singer & Singer, 1990). A super hero may be anyone the child sees as having great "power," anyone whom the child respects, or anyone the child wants to be. Thus, the exact type of super hero may vary. Young children may admire and want to be a mother, father, firefighter, Dora the Explorer, or Diego the Adventurer. Older children may pretend to be conventional super heroes like Spider-Man, Superman, or Luke Skywalker, or more everyday super heroes like an astronaut, a pilot, or a doctor. In play, super hero titles may be invented in relation to the other aspects of play. For example, a child suddenly may be acknowledged by self or the therapist as "super jumper," "the amazing frog boy," or "the incredible flying girl." Whom the child might experience as being a hero depends on the child's cognitive functioning, experience, and social context.

By playing a super hero, the child takes on these super hero qualities. The child becomes powerful and a helper to others. The child gets to imagine and experience the possibilities of what might be and what could be. This is very beneficial for children in general, who often inhabit a role of being helped and of being told what to do, and when to do things (Kelly-Byrne, 1989). For children with disabilities, who often experience greater loss of power over their own lives and who may suffer from low self-esteem, super hero play can be transformative (Parham, 1992). Through super hero play, the child is empowered to perform great feats or to help others. This can be a healing, coping strategy (Singer & Singer, 1990). Super hero play can be a beneficial alternative to destructive play in children who are angry (Livesay, 2007). Super hero play is consistent with our profession's valuing of intrinsic motivation and active engagement in occupation.

■ ADAPTING CHALLENGE AND COMPETITION

Challenge and competition are common elements in older children's play and thus are common considerations of an occupational therapist addressing play. As described in Chapter One, challenge and competition emerge as prominent aspects of play in middle childhood in the forms of games with rules, sports, and computer/video games (Florey & Greene, 2008). As a common form of play, pediatric clients may want to engage in challenging and competitive play and/or may need to develop skills in this form of play. Although it may be appropriate to include elements of challenge and competition in occupational therapy sessions, the use of these features is not always play. Many clients have difficulty tolerating losing, or even the possibility of losing, and gloat excessively with winning. Clients with anxiety, low self-esteem, or high awareness of their limitations avoid the mere attempt at a challenging task and prefer very easy tasks that they have mastered, where there is no risk of failure. For such children, occupational therapy sessions must include challenge and competition in carefully graded steps.

Challenge and Risk

When framed in a sequence of carefully graded steps, many pediatric clients respond well and enjoy the playful thrill that challenge can be. They enjoy the possibility of challenge in the face of some risk of defeat or failure. Even young children seek out and enjoy physical risk taking despite its "scariness" (Stephenson, 2003). Through limited risk experiences, children have described how they learn from their own mistakes (Christensen & Mikkelsen, 2008). Factors influencing a child's willingness to take risks versus avoiding risk taking include various child attributes (i.e., age, sex, experience, values, temperament), parent–family characteristics (i.e., socialization and teaching practices; parent modeling, style, and attributes; older sibling behavior and encouragement), and social-situational factors (peer risk taking and persuasion, media exposure, and convenience), as well as socioeconomics, culture, and neighborhoods (Morrongiello & Lasenby-Lessard, 2007).

Sometimes children with disabilities do not have the same enjoyment of challenge in play (Messier, Ferland, & Majnemer, 2008), and the occupational therapist must grade challenge so the client can play. Many children enjoy having these challenges framed in the context of other common social-cultural activities, such as advancing levels in a computer/video game, Olympics, circus/magic tricks, rodeo, *Survivor* television show, and so on. To build tolerance for challenge, first the occupational therapist suggests an easy *challenge*, a very simple action that the child can meet with ease. Perhaps, before increasing the demands, the therapist has the child repeat the success a few times to increase sense of mastery. Then the therapist keeps altering the activity slightly, notifying the child of the increasing challenge and including the child's ideas for increased challenges. The therapist playfully comments about how hard it is in general and elicits or offers positive comments about the child's potential for doing it—"This is pretty hard, but do you think you can do it? I think you can do it." If the activity has been carefully graded, by the time the child reaches the point of true challenge to his or her abilities, the child should have experienced repeated success in previous "challenge" attempts. This momentum increases the likelihood that the child will now attempt a true challenge and be willing to try again even if he or she fails. The occupational therapist has created a game where the challenge is fun because it is met successfully; where the child experiences satisfaction in meeting a challenge and begins to see him- or herself as a successful conqueror of challenges. The child has taken a risk and succeeded.

A note of caution is warranted here. Risk taking should be balanced with understanding and self-control to avoid truly dangerous, risky play that can injure the child (Morrongiello & Matheis, 2007b). Children must have an accurate understanding of the challenge in relation to their abilities and their vulnerability for injury (Morrongiello & Mathesis, 2007a, 2007b). The child must have some sense of fear of real dangers to be cautious and must be able to find excitement in safe activities (Cook, Peterson, & DiLillo, 1999; Morrongiello & Matheis, 2007b). As mentioned in Chapter One, cognitive-developmental play theorists assert that these skills can be developed in play. Occupational therapists can help children learn to play safely by assisting them in developing insight into their own abilities and an understanding of physical properties in the environment.

Competition

Competition involves a challenge between two or more people. This may be between the client and the therapist, family members, and/or peers. Although competitive games such as team sports are common in society, maintaining a healthy, balanced level of competition requires careful grading on the part of the occupational therapist. Competitive play has significant potential for aggression, anxiety, and hostility (Bay-Hinitz & Wilson, 2005). Sometimes pediatric clients become intensely competitive, throwing a tantrum when they lose and gloating when they win. These features make them unattractive playmates for competitive games, and without a playmate, children lose out on opportunities to play. Others may be so afraid of losing that they avoid this large category of play altogether. Issues of competition commonly arise when children are seen in group therapy sessions, and

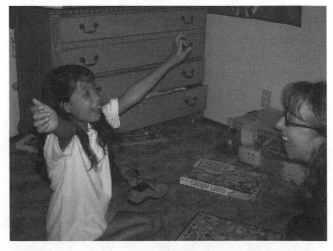

Winning a board game can be very exciting for a child, but the occupational therapist may need to grade competition to help the child learn to manage competition and tolerate losing as well.

Table 8-3   Strategies for Adapting Competitive Games

- Use games of personal challenge where the child plays the role of both winner and loser.

- Take turns in noncompetitive activities so that the child learns to tolerate sharing the joy and challenges of an activity with another person.

- Play games of pure chance—as long as the child can cognitively understand the explanation that it is just chance as to who wins or loses.

- Play games where no one wins or loses.

- Establish rules where points are awarded (only) for good sportsmanship, such as saying "good job" to teammate regardless of whether he or she is winning or losing.

- Restructure competitive games into cooperative games where all players work together to reach a common goal (Bay-Hinitz & Wilson, 2005).

- Control the relative amount/frequency of winning/losing to gradually stretch the child's ability to tolerate loss:

  – Alternate between winning and losing so that therapist and client essentially "take turns" with winning and losing

  – Have therapist get close to winning (creating a threat of loss for the client) but then lose

  – Have "a tie" where no one wins or loses

- Make a story or have a discussion about the process of playing games. Important points are that one person loses and one wins, how to handle both (good sportsmanship), and how it is more fun to play, regardless of winning or losing, than not to play at all.

- Model coping skills for losing and good sportsmanship.

group sessions provide natural opportunities to address competition.

Often, it is beneficial to start with games of personal challenge, where one competes against oneself. The client plays roles of both winner and loser. The occupational therapist can place greater emphasis on one or the other role depending on the child's needs. The occupational

therapist can emphasize how the client beat his or her last record, setting a new record. Even when the client does not beat his or her last record, that client still holds "the record" and may do better next time. **Table 8-3** lists additional ideas for adapting competitive games.

■ ADAPTING DANGER AND FEAR THEMES IN PLAY

The threat of danger and potential fear is a common theme in children's play. It can be exciting to watch out for dangerous animals (such as sharks, crocodiles, alligators, bears, lions, spiders, etc.), make-believe creatures (such as ghosts, monsters, and villains), and other threats (such as storms). This fear and threat of danger add an element of potential risk if the child makes a mistake, falls, or goes too close to where the danger is. Playing with fears is thought to help children feel more in control of their fears if they successfully express and manage them in play (Goetze, 1994; Mook, 1994; Singer & Singer, 1990). It adds drama and suspense to the story line or narrative structure of pretend play. The use of such potential dangers can be a playful technique for directing a child to do an activity in a certain way: "Stay on the path so the crocodiles don't get you!" It can also be used to help the child persevere through an extra challenge or error when he or she slips: "Oh no, it's quicksand, use all your muscles and you can get out." Overcoming danger or risk is what super heroes do, too.

These otherwise playful threats can also be the source of much fear and anxiety in some children. Young children are especially vulnerable because they may have difficulty recognizing and remembering that the danger is only pretend and not real (Singer & Singer, 1990). Other children do not have the emotional strength to handle such

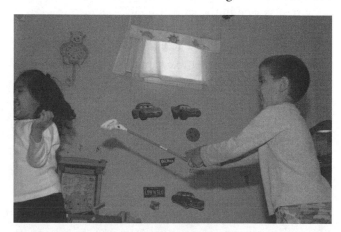

Playing with themes of pretend danger and fear with a toy shark can be very enjoyable for many children. However, for other children, such themes can be too threatening.

potential threats, which seem too real. Significant fear is associated with less willingness to take a risk and more protective behaviors in typical children of various ages (Cook et al., 1999; Morrongiello & Matheis, 2007b). Even if the child suggests it, he or she may have difficulty playing with this theme. Also, novelty itself can evoke some element of real fear and anxiety in children and impact the child's tolerance for pretend fear and danger. Therefore, the occupational therapist must carefully monitor the child when playing with themes of danger and fear, grade the activity carefully to ensure that the child is mostly successfully overcoming or escaping the "danger," and be ready to alter the activity and offer emotional support if needed.

■ DILEMMA OF UNDERGROUND PLAY THEMES

Play themes can be both helpful and challenging in therapy sessions. A number of play themes are common in Western society and easily can be used in therapy, such as delivering mail/valentines, being a super hero, making food, driving, trick-or-treating, or being an animal. However, as mentioned in Chapter Four, some common play themes can be disturbing to adults. For example, many adults feel uncomfortable when they see children playing themes related to aggression and violence (such as guns, jail, fighting, and war), death and dying, and bodily parts and functions. The therapist, parent, teacher, or others often prefer other types of play. This creates a therapeutic dilemma for the occupational therapist who wants to honor the child's play interests but also must contend with adult reservations about allowing such play. The occupational therapist must consider whether and how underground play themes can be incorporated into therapeutic activities, as seen in the case of Joey.

Therapists need to reflect on their own values and knowledge of play, as well as the values, needs, and interests of the child and other relevant adults (**Table 8-4**). The therapist must be careful not to push his or her own values onto the child, as discussed in Chapter Four. The therapist may want to consider information about the common presence of such themes in typical children's play, and the potential function of this play for the child's understanding of these difficult concepts. Occupational therapists can share this knowledge with parents, schools, or other relevant parties to help them make informed decisions. Even with this knowledge, a parent or institution may set rules against a certain type of play, thus setting the social-cultural boundaries for therapy. If a therapist feels strongly that such a type of play is important for a child,

Joey and the Dying Game

Joey was a 10-year-old with autism and developmental delays. He demonstrated difficulties with self-regulation of emotions and behavior. He was easily frustrated and upset, which usually resulted in aggression (hitting or grabbing others) and destruction of nearby physical property. Even when calm, he had significant difficulties with motor planning and grading force; he often accidentally hurt other people, broke objects, or ruined projects. He was being seen in the school occupational therapy room with a focus on play and sensory integration. He was easily frustrated and would try to stop or get out of therapeutic and daily life activities. During one session, he dropped to the ground and announced "I died." "Oh no, I'm going to miss you!" said the therapist. "Should I give you some medicine to help you feel better?" asked the therapist. "No!" replied Joey. "What should I do?" asked the therapist. "Bury me," said Joey. "Okay," said the therapist, "will this big pillow work?" "Yea," he replied. And she placed a large pillow on top of him and commented how she wished he would come back to play. After a moment, he pushed the pillow back and said, "I'm alive." "Yeah!" the therapist said. Joey then wanted the therapist to take a turn, and she did, with Joey carefully placing the pillow on top of her as she directed "gentle, just pretend." This became the basis for a more elaborate "dying game." First, they selected equipment that they could use together (determining adequate physical space for their two bodies). He would ask her, "Do you want to dance?" and hold out his hand. She put her hand in his and together they would get on a swing, being very attentive to maintain body space and be careful "like a gentleman." They would move the swing around in a "dance" and fall off together into a pillow, where he would say who was dead. The "alive" person would bury the "dead" one, carefully grading force. Then the "dead" person would come back to life, and the game was repeated. In the "dying game," Joey experienced sustained activity participation and learned to regulate his muscle force and emotions.

Learning Activity

Considering the case of Joey, what other ways could the occupational therapist have addressed the child's interest in underground play?

Table 8-4 Questions to Guide Clinical Reasoning With Underground Play Themes

- Which personal values are influencing my feelings about this child's play (positively or negatively)?

- What does the research evidence say about this type of play?

- Is it typical, common play?

- What are the potential benefits of this play?

- What are the potential risks (negative outcomes) of this play?

- What are the values of the child's family, friends, school, sociocultural group, etc. regarding this play?

- How does this form of play relate to the child's interests and needs?

- Does this child need help in learning to control and limit these themes to negotiate social environments?

- Does the child lack skills for other forms of play?

- Is this play in excess of the normal range and does it suggest that this child needs other adult assistance (psychology referral, social service/legal notification)?

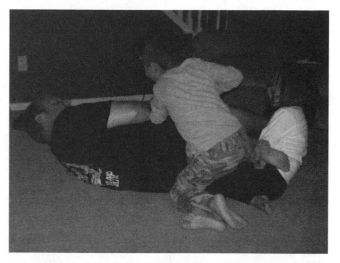

In some families, rough and tumble play may be acceptable for boys and girls, whereas other families may discourage or not allow aggressive-themed play for boys and/or girls.

the therapist may advocate for changes to these rules on behalf of the client.

Another consideration with such types of underground play themes is that typically, children also control and limit these play themes. They play a variety of play themes. They begin to understand when and with whom they can play such types of play—for example, 7- and 8-year-old boys learn to use "potty talk" in their games when out of earshot of adults. Children begin to recognize which objects can be thrown and hit, and which objects break. They learn to regulate force so as not to really hurt someone when play fighting. Often, it is adult feedback and rules that help them control and shape this form of play. When a child with a disability is learning to play, the therapist and adults in his or her life may have to play both roles of supporting and limiting or shaping this play. For example, the therapist may shape destructive forms of play away from "killing" and toward things that are socially acceptable to be destroyed or disciplined (such as litter, weeds, monsters, bad guys), or he or she may help the child enact a sequence of events related to aggression (such as rebuilding a building or giving "first

aid" for "injuries"). In some cases, the therapist may also have to set explicit limits/rules, especially where there is undue risk of injury to self or others or damage to property. Or, the occupational therapist may suggest alternative forms of play such as cooperative games that are inconsistent with aggression and allow the child to develop alternative social skills (Bay-Hinitz & Wilson, 2005).

Another clinical reasoning factor in underground play is assessing whether such play is within the range of typical play or whether it may be a sign that the child is struggling with an unusually strong emotional experience and needs adult help. For example, sometimes children begin to play with themes of death and dying when a pet or someone they know has died. If this theme comes up too often or with unusually strong real emotions shown, it may indicate that the child needs assistance with the grieving process, and the team psychologist or social worker should be consulted. A child who demonstrates real anger and aggression rather than play emotions may also need psychological intervention and a focus on cooperative play. Play therapy for children who need to focus on psychiatric problems such as antisocial behavior or who need to handle emotional stress from abuse, bereavement, or other trauma usually requires additional expertise and training to help the child express his or her feelings and cope with his or her situation through play activities (Blunden, 2001).

Sexual play is a specific example of underground play that requires the occupational therapist's clinical reasoning. Sexual play and behaviors are common in children but are often uncomfortable for adults. Typically, (developmentally) young children who have discovered their private body parts and how they may be different from others (e.g., presence or absence of penis/vagina, circumcised or uncircumcised penis) may start to talk about these factual discoveries, ask questions about body functions, engage in touching of or looking at their genitalia, and show interest in and curiosity about other aspects of sexuality (Larsson & Svedin, 2002; Sandnabba, Santtila, Wannas, & Krook, 2003). A wide variety of sexual behaviors is commonly observed in children, peaking at 3 to 5 years of development, but the behaviors at this age do not have the same cognitive and erotic meaning as adult sexuality (Pluhar, 2007). Conversely, the rare occurrence of sexual behaviors that imitate adult sexual behavior (oral–genital contact and insertion of object or body part into another child), and sexual preoccupation in a young child who does not demonstrate other preoccupations indicate that the child is less likely to have invented this behavior on his or her own and is more likely to have been exposed to sexual activity or to have been sexually abused; this is truly concerning when observed in children's play (Davies, Glaser, & Kossoff, 2000). Suspicious incidences or descriptions of sexual behavior must be reported to the authorities as required by law. For a good research-based resource on childhood sexual development and behaviors, the reader is referred to Pluhar (2007).

■ FAMILY PLAY

Often, family members may be included in playful therapeutic activities because this may be very beneficial for the pediatric client and the family as well. Chapter Six mentioned how occupational therapists may help others create a playful environment and learn how to support the child. This can be more challenging than it sounds.

First, the occupational therapist must monitor additional people beyond just the child. The occupational therapist must learn to divide attention and alternate different types of communication and interaction strategies for each individual. For example, it is not uncommon for parents focused on their child's success to be very directive to "make it happen." However, therapeutically, the goal is often for clients to do as much as possible on their own, and thus the occupational therapist may help the family develop a less directive approach. The family is typically taught the subtle ways of providing just enough prompting and support for the child to actively engage in the activity (Greenspan & Wieder, 1997; Lane & Mistrett, 2008; McConkey, 1994). Furthermore, the information the occupational therapist provides must be sensitive to

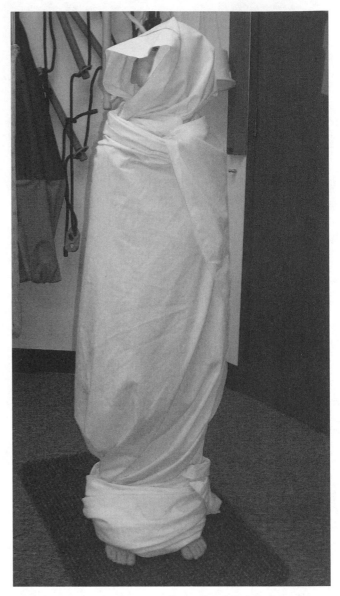

Being a mummy can be a new form of pretend play that allows the child to explore danger and fear themes. Although this can be especially culturally and temporally relevant at Halloween in some families, other families may object because of cultural values, religious beliefs, or personal opinions about appropriate play. The occupational therapist may discuss with the family the pros and cons of different forms of play for the child.

the other people present. For example, an explanation or direction to a parent can sound to the child like a criticism of the child's abilities.

Second, the family may have their own particular play routines (Primeau, 1998), interests, values, and opinions that do not immediately seem to support treatment outcomes or that may conflict with the therapist's personal or professional values. Families often rear their children and encourage and discourage play based on their interests, values, and cultural and socioeconomic backgrounds. For example, we have encountered families who do not want their children to play themes related to holidays they do not celebrate (Halloween costumes/characters, Santa Claus, Easter Bunny, birthday parties, etc.), aggressive play themes (guns, war, killing, etc.), dark or dangerous themes (e.g., monsters, etc.), television shows or videos (e.g., Disney, etc.), and processed foods (e.g., chips, hot dogs, etc.). Families may disapprove of the child's play interest as inappropriate or as a sign of disability. In fact, some families do not value play for their child or themselves, perhaps because they are so focused on the child's disability and are committed to working hard to minimize the effects of the disability (Knox, 1993), or they simply value hard work (McConkey, 1994). In such cases, occupational therapists may want to discuss why play in general or a specific play theme may be helpful therapeutically for the child and the parent–child relationship (Ferland, 2005). With a strong knowledge about play (see Chapters One and Two), the occupational therapist is prepared to engage in such health conversations. However, it is important that the occupational therapist not impose his or her values on the family (Hinojosa & Kramer, 2008). We must respect the family's culture, look for common ground, and focus on our therapeutic use of self to help the family facilitate the child's occupational performance (see Chapter Four).

■ PLAY IN OVERDRIVE:
TOO MUCH PLAYING AROUND?

Some children can become too involved with a particular aspect of an activity that is silly, fun, or interesting to them. Usually, this is when the child is very focused on one aspect of play and resists altering it or wants to repeat something to such a degree that therapy seems to be detoured. Children with attention deficit disorders often have difficulty attending to activities that are less than highly interesting. Other children may seek strong play experiences to avoid even the smallest challenge. These can be very stressful moments for the therapist, who may wonder if this detour from therapy may turn into total derailment. Although the entire goal of this book is facilitating play, we advocate facilitating play in therapy sessions for the *purpose* of therapeutic gains. When the child's engagement in play seems to be a roadblock for therapy, the occupational therapist's clinical reasoning is challenged. For example, a second-grader deciding to make a pencil into a puppet that makes silly sounds when the class is

writing quietly in their journals can be very aggravating for a school-based therapist. How can the occupational therapist keep play when it seems incompatible with therapy? It takes creative thinking to adapt these play activities based on sound activity analysis.

A Time and Place

Some children seem to find ways to be silly, make jokes, or play games all the time. Although this sounds like a trait this book might support, it may be problematic at certain times and places. When therapy is working on activities that require a child's serious focus, such as accuracy in writing or cutting, a client's playful approach can seem disruptive, with cuts and lines all over the paper. This playful behavior can also be disruptive during certain family and cultural events and in classrooms. At these times, the occupational therapist must make clinical judgments about the relative valuation of play, the setting, and work at hand, and the possibilities for creating activity adaptations. When the activity can be modified to meet the child's interests and the environmental demands, as discussed in Chapter Seven, this is often the preferred route. If no effective adaptations can be found, then sometimes the occupational therapist will have to set more explicit structure that allows for some play and some "work." Permitting some of this playfulness at first may be necessary to allow the child mastery over a new ability and encourage willingness to "buy in" to work, as the two cases of Sophia and Eddie illustrate.

Learning Activity

Consider the video cases from the treatment sessions on the DVD (you may want to review these again). In what ways did the occupational therapist:

- grade structure while balancing flexibility?
- grade challenge and risk?
- monitor danger and fear themes?
- manage a child's strong play drive in order to get the work of therapy done?

Obsessive Play

A child who is obsessed with one play form or theme may find this to be a wonderful play experience. A child may insist on exclusively playing cars, monsters, horses, or a particular character. However, the problems come when the child is so involved in this one play activity that he or she cannot adjust to play with other peers or tolerate changes that promote therapeutic goals. To both honor the child's play interests and promote therapeutic gains can be a challenge. Some of the strategies provided for extending limited play interests in Chapter Seven can be helpful. At other times, the occupational therapist is challenged to find as many ways as possible to combine the child's obsessive play focus with therapeutic goals. When one of the goals is to enhance the variety of play, the occupational therapist may find him- or herself brainstorming "101 ways to play _____ [the child's interest]." In other cases, where the goals are to build other

Sophia and Play Limits

Sophia was a 2 ½–year-old with developmental delays. She was being seen in a sensory integration clinic. Although she was socially interactive, she generally wandered around without clear engagement in play activities and became easily fearful during a range of therapy activities. The occupational therapist was using a sensory integration approach to optimize her arousal level, encouraging her to actively reach and throw various balls and toys into a bin. Sophia had played with these toys before and always recoiled when she saw the spider balls in the bin. She appeared genuinely scared and commented, "Ick." The occupational therapist always put them aside with an exaggerated "Ick" followed by a smile. During one session, Sophia asked for the spiders. Each time, she took the spider and waved it in the therapist's face, laughing as the therapist feigned exaggerated fear. At first, the occupational therapist was delighted with Sophia's management of her own fear and interest in playing a new game. But as it became clear that Sophia wanted to continue this game indefinitely, the occupational therapist realized that something would have to change to continue along the therapeutic path. So the occupational therapist set a limit, allowing Sophia to briefly scare the therapist and then, more seriously, having her let the spider go into a barrel because "Now it is time for the spider to go to bed." Although Sophia did not want to alter her play in this way, the therapist successfully encouraged her with an offer of getting another spider with which to do the same. It took some direction from the therapist, but Sophia did allow her spider game to be structured by the therapist.

Eddie and His Strong Play Drive

Eddie was a 4-year-old with delayed fine motor skills who avoided manipulating small toys, scissors, crayons, and other materials that would build his fine motor skills. He had a good sense of playfulness but resisted all activities that were even mildly challenging. He enjoyed a range of transportation vehicles such as cars, trucks, trains, motorcycles, and airplanes. The occupational therapist suggested a small wind-up train with open cart and round track. Eddie was immediately interested in watching the train go around and picking it up to look at it more closely. Then the occupational therapist brought out some small pegs as cargo to fill up the empty cart. Again, Eddie willingly helped fill up the cart. Although the occupational therapist was getting Eddie's playful engagement, she knew the activity still needed to be increased in challenge for it to be therapeutic for Eddie. She brought out some tongs, whose correct use would be therapeutic for Eddie's fine motor needs. She suggested that the tongs were a crane to load and unload the train. Eddie accepted this and began using the tongs with his whole hand in a more gross form than the finger precision the occupational therapist had envisioned. Nonetheless, she opted to let Eddie continue in this manner for a few minutes to build his comfort, acceptance, and interest in the activity before adding a new demand for precise use of the tongs. If she pushed the increased precision demand too fast, Eddie would stop the activity because he would no longer experience it as play. Because the occupational therapist waited and allowed Eddie to continue to engage in the playing that she had shaped, he was willing to tolerate her next demand, the true "work" demand.

Learning Activity

Considering the cases of Sophia and Eddie, in what other ways could the occupational therapist have changed play to promote therapeutic goals?

skills, the occupational therapist may help create a new play activity that combines the child's interest with therapeutic, skill-building activities, as illustrated in the case of Isabella.

Sometimes the process of expanding a very particular play focus can take time and occurs gradually. Vivian Paley, a preschool teacher, detailed this process for Jason, one of her students, over the course of a school year (Paley, 1990). Jason had an obsessive and solitary play interest of pretending to be a helicopter and refusing to let others enter his play. With the support from his teachers and the other students, Jason gradually tolerated interaction with others as a "helicopter" and eventually learned to "park" his helicopter to play other themes as well. Kluth and Schwarz (2008) have provided a number of other strategies for including obsessive interests in educational programs.

Isabella, Presidents, and Geography

Isabella was a bright kindergartner with an anxiety disorder who had developed a strong interest in information related to American presidents and world geography. She loved to talk about recent knowledge she had gained in these areas. Occupational therapy was focused on building self-confidence, balance, bilateral coordination, and timing for greater participation at recess, and increased visual-spatial constructional skills for improved ability to draw, write, and make class projects. She was being seen in a school therapy room using a sensory integration approach. Her occupational therapist suggested that they play world traveling. Isabella asked if they could play American presidents traveling the world, and her occupational therapist agreed. To work on gross motor skills, they used different equipment to represent different countries or modes of traveling to each location. Isabella was quick to identify countries to start at and where to travel to, but despite her studied knowledge of the world, she was unable to identify their relative locations and distances. Her occupational therapist borrowed a world map from a teacher so that Isabella could look at the location of each country before making the trip on suspended equipment. In this way, the occupational therapist helped Isabella to work on spatial orientation through determining direction and estimating relative spatial distance to determine long, medium, and short trips.

Learning Activity

Considering the case of Isabella, in what other way could the occupational therapist have addressed Isabella's needs and strong interests in play?

Learning Activity

Occupational therapists often must come up with many different ways to incorporate a child's narrow interests. These interests can vary dramatically. Some are more common than others. Nonetheless, practicing your ability to quickly identify multiple ways of integrating different interests with therapeutic goals will help you be more efficient in the real time of actual treatment sessions.

How many different activities can you think of for each of the following sample interests? (Give yourself 2 minutes for each interest.)

- cars
- Star Wars
- Barbie dolls
- Civil War
- monsters
- babies

■ ADOLESCENT PLAY IN OCCUPATIONAL THERAPY

When working with adolescents, occupational therapists may find it difficult to incorporate play because many forms of play can be too juvenile, and yet play is still relevant through adulthood. Key ways of incorporating play with an adolescent client include using sports, peer interaction, video games, board/card games, humor, and balancing play and healthy leisure.

As mentioned in Chapter One, sports activities continue as a typical play interest of adolescents. Both directly playing and following sports are common. In occupational therapy with adolescents, sports-based themes and gross motor games with rules and competition are used frequently. Often, these are done in the context of groups with other peers.

Video games are a common play interest in developed countries, and thus occupational therapy with adolescents must often consider the use of video games and participation in video games. In their review of the literature, Gooch and Living (2004) recommended the use of video games with adolescents in occupational therapy because they can promote feelings of mastery and competence, and they are age appropriate, normalizing, and culturally appropriate. Video games can be socially appealing to adolescents because they allow teens the opportunity to engage in competitive play even if they do not excel at sports, offer a means for companionship when playing in a group, and provide social capital for discussion topics and relating to peers (Raney, Smith, & Baker, 2006). Moderate use of video games appears to be generally safe in health care and poses no long-term health problems (Griffiths, 2005); however, excessive use of media in general (including video games) has been associated with negative health outcomes, including obesity and smoking in adolescents (Common Sense Media, 2008). To minimize negative effects on health, the American Academy of Pediatrics (2001) recommends a daily limit of 2 hours' total media use (including video games and television). Helping to achieve a healthy balanced use of media may be a role for occupational therapy.

Another form of play activity that can span childhood through adolescence to adulthood is table-top games such as board games and card games. Board games have been used to teach and practice daily living skills, such as social, money management, and emergency-preparedness skills for

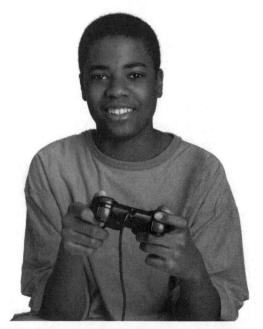

As a common play interest for adolescents, video games may be considered in occupational therapy with adolescents.

individuals with developmental disabilities (Hurff, 1981) and to increase standing tolerance (Hoppes, 1997). To establish reasonable expectations for successful performance on a game, occupational therapists and researchers can record the performance of a sample of adolescents as Neistadt, McAuley, Zecha, and Shannon (1993) did for the game Hi-Q with a convenience sample of 18 adults.

Humor becomes more complex with development, and it is commonly associated with playfulness into adulthood (Barnett, 2007; Guitard, Ferland, & Dutil, 2005). It is a common mode of "hanging out" with friends. As mentioned in Chapter Four, humor can be risky because there are individual and cultural differences in humor, and sometimes humor for one person is offensive to another. This is especially true in adolescence as humor becomes more complex. Usually, it is best to use humor that involves a play on words or saying/doing the opposite of what you actually mean while avoiding humor that the client may perceive as teasing or belittling. A young teenager may even enjoy "opposite day," where both client and therapist must say the opposite of what they mean (e.g., "do" for "don't," etc.); the opposites can be funny in themselves, and it can be amusing when one person forgets and the other does the opposite of what was expected. When the adolescent asks "Why do I have to do this?" the occupational therapist may be able to say jokingly, "because I am so mean." Certainly, this level of humor requires a client's cognitive understanding and emotional tolerance to see something as funny and not real.

Adolescents often like to entertain extreme ideas without concern for the reality that makes these ideas virtually impossible: for example, "Wouldn't it be cool if I could jump off the building with my bike and land without getting hurt or close my eyes and wish my homework done?" and so on. Although verbalizing such daydreaming fantasies can be an extension of pretend play or humor, it is important to make sure the adolescent also understands the reality that such ideas cannot be acted on because adolescents tend not to recognize their own mortality and may minimize the long-term consequences of their actions. As mentioned in Chapter One, as adolescents become more independent in making decisions about how to spend their time, balancing play with other activities and establishing healthy leisure pursuits are common developmental challenges that may continue into adulthood (Poulsen & Ziviani, 2006; Spencer, 1989). Consequently, this is also a key area for occupational therapy to address with this population.

■ CONCLUSION

In this chapter, we presented the reader with a number of examples of specific challenges that may confront the occupational therapist who uses play in intervention. Factors to consider and examples of analyzing, grading, and modifying activities were offered. As interesting as these situations are, you will certainly encounter others that will be both similar and different in your practice. As research on play in occupational therapy continues, more research likely will be available to assist you in your clinical reasoning. Along the way, we hope that you will find these to be attainable challenges that are also enjoyable and motivating for you to engage in creatively. Have fun!

Appendix 8-1

Suggested Resources on Creating Therapeutic Stories

Baltazar, A., & Bax, B. E. (2004). Writing social stories for the child with sensory integration dysfunction: An introductory resource and guide for therapists, teachers, and parents. *Sensory Integration Special Interest Section Quarterly, 27*(1), 1–3.

Fazio, L. S. (2008). Storytelling, storymaking, and fantasy play. In L. D. Parham & L.S. Fazio (Eds.), *Play in occupational therapy for children* (2nd ed., pp. 427–443). St. Louis, MO: Mosby Elsevier.

Gray, C. (2000). *The new social story book.* Arlington, TX: Future Horizons.

Levine, K., & Chedd, N. (2007). *Replays: Using play to enhance emotional and behavioral development for children with autism spectrum disorders.* London: Jessica Kingsley.

Marr, D., & Nackley, V. (2007). Writing your own sensory stories. *OT Practice, 12*(11), 15–19.

Sensory Stories (*www.sensorystories.com*) is a fee-based Web application to assist therapists in writing sensory stories for clients.

Speakingofspeech.com (*http://www.speakingofspeech.com/Materials_Exchange.html*) has a variety of examples of therapeutic stories that can be downloaded free of charge to use with clients.

The Gray Center for Social Learning and Understanding (*www.thegraycenter.org*) provides information on Social Stories.

Section Four
Additional Considerations

9

Examining the Evidence

After completing this chapter, the reader will

1. Describe the research related to play assessment, activity analysis, playful therapeutic use of self, and play interventions.

2. Discuss the limitations and needs of current research related to play in pediatric occupational therapy.

> *In our play we reveal what kind of people we are.*
> —Ovid

This book has provided a foundation of knowledge, a vision, and opportunities for developing skills in activity analysis and the creative use of play in pediatric occupational therapy. This process is advocated to develop a therapeutic relationship and to provide meaningful client-centered therapeutic interventions and outcomes. Chapters One through Four provided the relevant descriptive research that provides a foundation for play-based occupational therapy. In this chapter, we will turn to examining additional research to establish the state of evidence related to therapeutic effectiveness. Although many aspects of play-based occupational therapy are supported by research, far more research is needed to establish effectiveness and to determine the relative benefit of different strategies for a wide variety of client populations. This chapter summarizes and discusses key research that supports the assessment, intervention, and therapeutic use of self strategies described in this book, as well as research limitations and opportunities for future research.

■ PLAY ASSESSMENT AND ACTIVITY ANALYSIS

Chapter Three covered formal and informal play assessment, including activity analysis and goal writing for play. In considering this knowledge base, the following questions arise: What evidence supports the evaluation of play, the use of specific assessment methods for the examination of play, and the use of the tool of activity analysis? What is known about goal writing and its influence on our practice?

There is a growing body of work devoted to the assessment of playfulness and play preferences. The research on assessing playfulness is thoroughly described elsewhere (Skard & Bundy, 2008). The Test of Playfulness is a reliable and valid tool that has been used in multiple studies. A few studies described in Chapter Three suggest that children can discuss the meaning of their play and the implications of specific characteristics of play in determining their play preferences. Additionally, Spitzer's research (2003a, 2003b), described in Chapter Three, indicates that therapists can determine the meaning of children's play choices, even for children without the ability to communicate.

Sadly, there is just one study (Couch, Deitz, & Kanny, 1998) to date that examines the practices of occupational therapists in terms of their typical use of play assessments and their inclusion of play as an area in their full evaluation. This study found that therapists were not routinely evaluating play nor including play in their goal writing or specific intervention plans, which suggested the need for this book. Now, more than 10 years later, it is important to determine if things have changed in response to the literature on play in the past decade. Additionally, an important question is, if we increase the use of play assessments in our practice, will we, in turn, increase the likelihood of the inclusion of play goals to guide our intervention? Research would be helpful to answer the question of whether occupational therapists who more frequently include play goals also focus more often on play and become more playful. What would the long-term impact of this be on our practice and our outcomes?

There has been little research completed on the process of activity analysis, either in how students learn it, in how therapists use it, or in how effective it is in helping therapists provide interventions. Llorens, in an endeavor to make activity analysis more reliable and valid, examined features of activity analysis in a group of 80 occupational therapy students and 47 occupational therapists (Llorens, 1973, 1986, 1993). She found 80% or better agreement among raters who participated in and completed the five different activities for many of the specific rating factors. She also found agreement between raters who participated in and completed the activity and those who observed the activity. However, agreement between participants and observers was greater for the factors that were more clearly visible, such as motions, and less likely for factors that were invisible, such as feelings.

There are many areas for future investigation on activity analysis that would provide valuable information to our profession. If we believe, as occupational therapists, that activity analysis is an important tool of our profession, we should demonstrate that after training and experience, occupational therapists are better able to use this tool than those who are untrained. To better understand how to facilitate this process in our students and novice therapists, we must also examine how this skill develops over time. Finally, it might be interesting to determine if other professionals and our clients consider this a skill and regard occupational therapists as having particular skill in this area. In our efforts to promote occupational therapy in the greater community, we should promote recognition of our skill in this area by consumers and other professionals.

■ PLAYFUL THERAPEUTIC USE OF SELF

The research on playful therapeutic use of self is drawn primarily from the occupational therapy literature on therapeutic use of self and from interdisciplinary research on adult–child play. Chapter Four reported the extensive research describing key elements that are used in therapeutic use of self and adult–child play. Here we present additional research on the outcomes of therapeutic use of self and the relationship of adult–child play to children's play

participation and development. Although this research supports the strategies detailed in Chapter Four, these bodies of descriptive and correlational research have limitations with regard to causality. Given the limitations of the research, clinical experience can supplement this research base, and clinical judgment is required in determining which strategies are a good match for individual children. We hope that future research will improve our clinical reasoning for playful therapeutic use of self in pediatric occupational therapy.

The occupational therapy literature asserts that therapeutic use of self is a central tool of effective practice (Devereaux, 1985; Price, 2009; Peloquin, 1990; Schwartzberg, 1993; Yerxa, 1967) that enables positive outcomes. As described in Chapter Four, practicing occupational therapists also consistently report that therapeutic use of self and therapeutic relationships influence positive outcomes (Cole & McLean, 2003; Gahnstrom-Strandqvist, Tham, Josephsson, & Borell, 2000; Hasselkus & Dickie, 1994; Rosa & Hasselkus, 1996; Taylor, Lee, Kielhofner, & Ketkar, 2009). Research supports that client-centered practices (focused on client goals) lead to improved client satisfaction and outcomes (Law, 1998). For example, Darragh, Sample, and Krieger (2001) studied client perceived intervention effectiveness among adults with brain injury. They found that client reports of treatment effectiveness were associated with practitioner roles such as advocate, friend, mentor, and team member, and practitioner characteristics such as being a clear and honest communicator, supportive, respectful, a good listener, and understanding. Palmadottir's (2003) research also found that the therapist–client relationship had a significant impact on adult rehabilitation clients' descriptions of occupational therapy's impact on their lives. In this study, clients described occupational therapy as a having a strong positive impact when the therapist–client relationship was characterized by trust and respect. Clients experienced a positive relationship if the occupational therapist demonstrated a caring attitude by paying attention to their feelings and showing interest in them (Palmadottir, 2006). Taylor and Peloquin (2008) found that therapeutic relationships in occupational therapy were consistently associated with positive outcomes. Even for medical conditions such as irritable bowel syndrome, a warm and supportive patient–physician relationship was found to promote clinical patient improvements (Kaptchuk et al., 2008). The two most significant limitations in this body of research are that (1) most of these studies are with adult clients, and (2) they are not experimental studies in occupational therapy.

Given the limitations of the research on therapeutic use of self, we also based Chapter Four on related research on the relationship between adult–child interaction and children's play, which indicates that adult interaction can influence children's play. Toddlers demonstrated more complex play when playing with their mothers than when playing by themselves (Fiese, 1990). Children between the ages of 12 months and 48 months demonstrated longer pretend play episodes with their mother than when playing by themselves (Haight & Miller, 1992). Infants demonstrated more complexity and engagement in play when their mothers interacted with them than when their mothers were merely present and not interactive (Sorce & Emde, 1981). Both verbal commentary and action by mothers were associated with increased level and length of play in toddlers (Slade, 1987). When mothers were given feedback and encouraged to use interactive strategies more frequently, their 1-year-olds demonstrated more competent play than 1-year-olds whose mothers were not given feedback or encouragement (Belsky, Goode, & Most, 1980). In children aged 12 to 47 months, symbolic play was correlated with encouraging mother interactions (demonstrating or offering toys or ideas) and negatively correlated with correcting mother interactions; however, the opposite trend was revealed for nonsymbolic play, which was correlated with correcting mother interactions and negatively correlated with encouraging mother interactions (Noll & Harding, 2003).

Similar increases in children's play have been associated with caregiver interaction for children with disabilities. Play was positively associated with caregiver interaction for 12-month-olds who were born premature (Lawson, Parrinello, & Ruff, 1992) and in 10- to 38-month-olds who were institutionalized (Daunhauer, Coster, Tickle-Degnen, & Cermak, 2007). Daunhauer et al. (2007) specifically found correlations in play engagement with caregivers who provided more structure, assistance, direction, and encouragement. Playfulness in young children with motor delay has been associated with both the child's developmental abilities and the parents' responsiveness (Chiarello, Huntington, & Bundy, 2006). Evans and Meyer (1999) found that modifying adult interactions to use social and playful communication strategies was effective in decreasing negative behaviors in a 3-year-old with Rett syndrome. Nadel, Martini, Field, Escalona, and Lundy (2008) found that children with autism aged 3 to 7 years looked at, approached, and touched adults more frequently when the adult more often looked at the child, smiled at the child, moved toward the child, had relaxed body tone, made sounds, imitated the child, and was playful. In sum, these research findings suggest that adult–child play facilitates children's play in typically developing infants and toddlers and in children with disabilities; however, the research is predominantly correlational. Additional research is also needed to better identify which interaction strategies build play, especially in children with different disabilities, with various developmental needs, and in a variety of socioeconomic and cultural backgrounds.

Hinojosa (2007) argued that innovation in occupational therapy requires concentrated study of therapeutic use of self and professional relationships. If therapeutic use of self is the essence of practice, then it is a valid pursuit to develop research that explores and justifies this caring process (Gilfoyle, 1980). We need more studies on therapeutic use of self with children and experimental studies that measure actual practices and dependent outcome variables (Table 9-1). Although it may be difficult to quantify and conclusively study such an artistic process, certainly more research is possible and desirable.

■ INTERVENTION EFFECTIVENESS

Throughout Section Three of this book, we presented a number of methods, forms, and examples of selecting, grading, and modifying play activities in pediatric occupational therapy. Some of these come from established literature and developmental descriptive research as noted in Chapters One and Two, and others are based on our experiences applying traditional activity analysis and clinical reasoning in pediatrics. This empirically informed intervention begs additional evidence of therapeutic effectiveness. Here we review the efficacy research on play, both as a means for improving other skills in occupational therapy and as an outcome of intervention itself.

Table 9-1   Research Questions for Future Studies of Playful Therapeutic Use of Self in Pediatric Occupational Therapy

- Is playful therapeutic use of self an effective intervention tool with children?
- Which strategies are more effective in general and for which specific groups of children?
- What factors are related to the development of more playful practitioners?
- Can classroom professors or fieldwork educators promote playfulness as an outcome in occupational therapists through their educational activities?

Play as Modality for Skill Building

Research studies have found play to be an effective modality in occupational therapy for improving visual-motor skills, fine motor skills, gross motor skills, social-emotional development, cognitive development, language, activities of daily living, functional back and neck extension, and behavior in children with various disabilities and parent self-concept and pleasure (Case-Smith, 2000; Esdaile, 1996; Olson, Heaney, & Soppas-Hoffman, 1989; Sakemiller & Nelson, 1998; Sparling, Walker, & Singdahlsen, 1984). This is consistent with research outside our profession that also found play to be an effective modality for promoting development of various skills, behavior, and mental health in children with different disabilities and needs (Bratton & Ray, 2000; Bratton, Ray, Rhine, & Jones, 2005; DeGangi, Wietlisbach, Goodin, & Scheiner, 1993; Fall, Navelski, & Welch, 2002; Leister, Langenbrunner, & Walker, 1995; Moore & Russ, 2006; Reddy, Files-Hall, & Schaefer, 2005; Skellenger & Hill, 1994).

Using play as a modality for improving other skills also is supported by research that indicates greater participation and intrinsic motivation with play activities than work activities. For example, Glynn's (1994) research with adults indicated that framing an activity as play rather than work increases intrinsic motivation and focus on the process rather than the product. This research is consistent with occupational therapists' reports that play is important in motivating and positively reinforcing children (Couch et al., 1998). Hanley, Cammilleri, Tiger, and Ingvarsson (2007) found that most preschool children did not select instructional stations over various types of play stations available in their classroom. Heal and Hanley (2007) found that preschool children selected a play-oriented activity over three different teaching contexts (highly preferred materials, highly preferred edible items for correct responding, and less preferred teaching materials). Such research on the positive outcomes of including play supports the philosophy of the play strategies advocated in this book. This research supports that play activities are more likely to elicit children's active participation in occupational therapy.

Whether play is more effective than other interventions is less clear. DeGangi et al.'s (1993) study suggests that play in occupational therapy is more effective in promoting fine motor skills but not other skills. Specifically, they compared a child-initiated play approach with a therapist-directed, structured sensorimotor approach with preschoolers with sensorimotor dysfunction. They found that structured sensorimotor therapy was more useful than child-centered therapy in promoting gross motor skills, functional abilities, and sensory integrative functions. The child-centered play approach was better at promoting fine motor skills. There were no differences between the two approaches for gains in play, attention, and behavior, and the authors suggest that these outcomes may have been related to an interaction of the approach with other variables, such as temperament, attentional abilities, family stress, severity of sensorimotor delay, and past intervention. Similarly, Case-Smith's (2000) study suggested that including play in occupational therapy may be more effective for fine motor and visual-motor skill development than not including play. Specifically, she followed 44 preschool-age children with fine motor delays who received occupational therapy services, using pretest and posttest measures and collected data on the format and intervention activities of each occupational therapy session. She found that positive visual-motor outcomes were associated with the percent of sessions focused on play goals and that positive fine motor outcomes were associated with the therapists' emphasis on play and peer interaction goals; however, functional self-care outcomes were not associated with play. This is consistent with a research study outside our profession (Howard, Miles, & Griffith, 2004, as cited in Howard, Jenvey, & Hill, 2006), in which the use of playful practice was significantly more effective than formal practice in clients' ability to complete a jigsaw puzzle. Another research study from outside our profession (Bernard-Opitz, Ing, & Kong, 2004) found that behavioral discrete trial training was more effective at increasing compliance than was a play-based intervention for young children with autism. Given that compliance is related to another person's direction, rule, or standard, it may not be as compatible with play outcomes, which are intrinsically motivated, and learning outcomes, which require an active self to acquire knowledge and skills. As described in this book, compliance with work activities can be reframed to be more playlike in occupational therapy and, if researched in this way, might have differing results for "compliance." Interestingly, in the Bernard-Opitz et al. (2004) study, the behavioral intervention was even more effective at increasing compliance when immediately preceded by the play intervention than when following it. This supports a common strategy used in many pediatric occupational therapy sessions, especially using a sensory integration approach, that start with play and then follow with more work-oriented activities at the end. This research suggests that the relationship between play-based intervention and work compliance may be complicated and warrants further study.

Play as Outcome of Occupational Therapy Intervention: Focus on Occupation

A small body of research has also examined the effectiveness of occupational therapy on play outcomes. Both modifications and direct intervention have been studied.

Several studies found that modifying the play context can have a positive impact on play skills and participation in children with disabilities. Schaaf and Mulrooney (1989) found that occupational therapy focused on the family yielded positive changes in play participation and motor skills for five young children. Hanzlik (1989) compared occupational therapy focused on 1 hour of parent training/instruction with 1 hour of a neurodevelopmental treatment approach for children aged 8 to 32 months with cerebral palsy. Mothers in the experimental group were instructed individually with their children in how to decrease constant physical contact and directiveness and increase positive initiations, responses, and praise with their children. Infants in the experimental parent training group engaged in more voluntary responsiveness and less physically directed compliance than those in the neurodevelopmental treatment control group. Additionally, mothers in the experimental group engaged in less directive physical guidance and contact and more positive initiations, responses, and face-to-face contact and used more adaptive seating than mothers in the control group. Such changes in child and mother behavior are more consistent with promoting play; however, the increases in the amount of independent play in the experimental group did not differ significantly from the neurodevelopmental treatment control group. In a follow-up study (Okimoto, Bundy, & Hanzlik, 2000), the videotapes from Hanzlik's study were used to rate playfulness of the children. Playfulness did increase significantly in the children who received the parent training intervention; however, this increase was not significantly higher than for those children who received the neurodevelopmental treatment approach. O'Brien et al. (1998) found that positioning equipment increased the play skills of physically impaired children as measured by parent report. Tanta, Deitz, White, and Billingsley (2005) found that preschool-age children with play delays generally showed more initiation and response to initiation during play when paired with a peer with higher developmental play skills than with a peer who had lower developmental play skills. Bundy et al. (2008) found that 20 typically developing 5- to 7-year-old children were significantly more playful after the introduction of various novel materials on the playground over the course of 11 weeks. Qualitative descriptions from the teachers also indicated that these children's play had become more active, creative, and social.

A few preliminary studies suggest that direct occupational therapy intervention with children also may have a positive impact on promoting play. In 1987, Schaaf, Merrill, and Kinsella conducted a single case study with a child who received occupational therapy using a sensory integration approach, which typically includes play. Based on qualitative assessment, they reported that the child's object play, parallel play, and exploratory play increased. In 1990, Schaaf conducted a single case study with a 5-year-old who received occupational therapy using a sensory integration approach. The child showed improvements in increased imaginative play, participation in tactile-based play activities, interaction with others, and time/attention in play. In 2000, O'Brien et al. conducted a pretest and posttest experimental study of the effectiveness of occupational therapy on increasing play skills and playfulness. The participants in each group were four children aged 4 to 6 years with no known physical impairments but difficulty playing per parent report. They had diagnoses of autism, communication disorder, and pervasive developmental disorder. The experimental group received occupational therapy 1 hour per week for 10 weeks, with a focus on increasing play skills and playfulness; home activity suggestions were included. The control group did not receive occupational therapy but did receive a home activity program. Two children in the treatment group made improvements in playfulness, and one also made improvements in play skills. They were the ones who attended the most sessions (eight to nine sessions). However, two children in the control group also made increases in playfulness. It is important to note that the children in the control group were receiving other therapeutic interventions, and the control and treatment groups were not matched groups. Studies of the Denver Model interdisciplinary program, which includes occupational therapy and focuses on play, found significant improvements in symbolic play skills as well as development for young children with autism and other developmental disabilities (Rogers, 2005). These studies are limited in effect size, sample size, population, age, and methodological standards. Further research is needed to better support the effectiveness of occupational therapy on promoting play skills and participation.

Play as an Outcome of Other Interventions

Findings within the field of occupational therapy are similar to the results found in studies of other interventions. For example, a meta-analysis of play therapy found that including parents in play therapy produced the largest effects of therapy (Bratton et al., 2005). Furthermore, the research on parent–child play (as reviewed earlier) also indicates that various adult interactions can promote play in young children. Educational staff reported that environmental changes on the playground have also been effective in increasing active, imaginative, constructive, and cooperative social play on the playground in general, and for a broader range of children with intellectual and physical disabilities (Bell & Dyment, 2006).

A significant body of research indicates that children with disabilities can learn to participate in higher level or more age-appropriate play activities through targeted intervention. For example, studies found adult prompting (gestures, verbal, physical) and praise/reinforcement to be effective in expanding the level of toy play (DiCarlo, Reid, & Stricklin, 2003; Incze, n.d.; Lifter, Ellis, Cannon, & Anderson, 2005; Malone & Langone, 1999), pretend/symbolic play (DiCarlo & Reid, 2004; Kasari, Freeman, & Paparella, 2006; Kim, Lombardino, Rothman, & Vinson, 1989), and social play (Kohl & Beckman, 1990) in children with disabilities. Modeling of scripted ways to play that children observe has also been effective in promoting targeted play (Nevile & Bachor, 2002; Thomas & Smith, 2004). Stories that explain and describe social behavior have also been supported as effective strategies for teaching play skills for children with autism (Barry & Burlew, 2004). It is important to note that much of this research on teaching play skills to children with disabilities involved primarily children with autism, younger children, and small sample sizes; lacked family and demographic diversity; and seldom employed control groups.

Outcomes of Interventions Using Child's Interests

Several studies support that including child choice, preference, or interest can be an effective strategy for promoting engagement in toy play and social play in children with autism (Baker, Koegel, & Koegel, 1998; Koegel, Dyer, & Bell, 1987; Reinhartsen, Garfinkle, & Wolery, 2002). Reinhartsen et al. (2002) also found that child choice resulted in more engaged time with toys for all three 2-year-old boys and fewer problematic behaviors for two of them. Although not specifically addressing play, Renninger (1990) compared the use of objects that were of greatest interest and objects that were not of interest during free play in visual attention and memory tasks for 3-year-olds and found that the children did significantly better when the objects of personal interest were used. Similarly, Vismara and Lyons's (2007) research found that when the child's individual perseverative or highly preferred interest was

included as a reinforcer in a behavioral program (pivotal response training), the social interactions of three children with autism increased without directly targeting those social interactions. Such research on the positive outcomes of including children's interests supports the play approach described and advocated throughout this book.

■ EFFECTIVENESS RESEARCH: IMPLICATIONS FOR OCCUPATIONAL THERAPY

Although the research presented in the preceding section is of relevance to and supports our practice, occupational therapy needs more research that examines the outcome of play as an occupation, not just an age-appropriate activity. It is important to recognize that the research generally supports play as a modality for promoting skills and development in play and other areas. But is intervention that is focused on play skills *play*? We cannot assume that all play interventions involve play as an occupation because "many of the more structured, behaviorally-based play interventions are far too adult-directed, goal-oriented, and involuntary to be deemed true play" (Mastrangelo, 2009, p. 14). Another key question for occupational therapists is: Does a play skills program yield an outcome of increased participation in *play* as an occupation? Research is still needed that supports how intervention can promote engagement in play as an occupation (for example, as defined in Chapter Two). Even if occupational therapists teach a child to engage in a behavior and they do so, the question remains as to whether it is play. That is, is it enjoyable? Is it an attainable challenge? Is it self-selected? Furthermore, what is the impact on the health of the child and family? This is the research we need in pediatric occupational therapy if we as occupational therapists intend to support our values and philosophy about play and playfulness with the effectiveness of real outcomes.

Effectiveness of Different Strategies

In addition to needing research that demonstrates effectiveness, occupational therapists need research that examines different strategies within therapy to determine the most efficient methods for practice. We need to know which strategies are most effective for which clients and for which outcomes (play skills, play as an occupation, and inclusive play participation). Few comparison studies exist.

In one study (Kok, Kong, & Bernard-Opitz, 2002), the effect of a structured play approach of explicit teaching and mass trials was compared with a facilitated play approach of incidental teaching for eight preschoolers with autism. In both conditions, appropriate play and communication increased. However, their results suggested that the structured approach was more effective for children with lower mental age, less speech and language, and very limited social interaction, whereas the facilitated approach was more effective for children with a higher mental age who were verbal and had better social abilities. Thus, different strategies may be more effective for different children.

Reid's (2004) study is another good example of this type of comparative research. She examined the differential impact of different virtual reality play sessions on playfulness for 13 children aged 8 to 13 years with cerebral palsy. Participants were randomly assigned to three different virtual reality play formats during each session. The participants' playfulness varied with the different virtual reality play environment forms. The forms that produced the highest playfulness ratings allowed more creativity, persistence with the task, pleasure, and degree of control. The two forms that did not appear to foster playfulness were more unpredictable and frustrating for participants. The findings of Reid's study are consistent with the general approach for grading play activities presented in this book. Far more studies are needed to explicate the strategies that are most effective for promoting play in pediatric clients with different needs, sociocultural backgrounds, and disabilities, and at different points in development.

Future Research Needs

Our profession needs a series of strong effectiveness studies to answer a range of questions about play in occupational therapy with clients of different ages, disabilities, needs, and cultural and socioeconomic backgrounds (**Table 9-2**). It is equally important that the methods are rigorous, with pretest and posttest measures, adequate sample size, and randomized and appropriately matched control subjects. Given the definitional challenges of play presented in Chapter One, quality studies will also have to address the same challenge of fidelity as have researchers in sensory integration (Parham et al., 2007) in order to ensure that play elements are included (Bundy, 1993). Intervention procedures must be designed with a documented intervention protocol and a means of verifying fidelity to the planned procedures in order to ensure that play elements are included. Play researchers may want to follow the lead of sensory integration researchers who are collaborating with

Table 9-2   Clinical and Research Questions on Effectiveness of Play-Based Occupational Therapy

- Is occupational therapy effective in increasing playfulness and play participation for children with different disabilities and needs, across different ages and diverse backgrounds, for different types of play?

- Which strategies are more effective in general and for which specific children?

- How does a play-based approach impact an occupational therapist's practice (i.e., job satisfaction, burnout, efficacy, etc.)?

- Does including peers and family members in play-based occupational therapy have a positive impact on peers and family members?

- Is play-based occupational therapy more effective than a skill-based approach for increasing children's participation in other (nonplay) activities such as self-care and handwriting?

- Is a play-based approach more effective than a skill-based approach for promoting health and well-being in pediatric clients?

each other to build a comprehensive research base for a similarly highly individualized intervention. This research is needed to support our belief that occupational therapists can improve play and playfulness through occupational therapy and that this improvement will lead to important benefits for the child and family. These hypotheses must be examined with further experimental research.

■ CONCLUSION

The number of studies reviewed in this chapter and the literature cited throughout this book illustrate the foundation of evidence for the strategies and approach that we advocate. There is research to support assessing play, using a playful therapeutic use of self, and intervening with play. However, it is important to recognize that this research has significant limitations. Many questions remain unanswered. Many hypotheses remain untested. It is important to recognize the current state of research evidence as you make clinical decisions. Clinically, such gaps in knowledge must be filled in by clinical judgment and experience. This book has supplemented the research gap with examples from our decades of collective pediatric clinical experience. We hope that you will draw on the examples of clinical reasoning that fill this book to assist you in making challenging clinical decisions. We also hope that, by identifying future research needs, others will be inspired to add to this evidence base so we all can improve our ability to make therapeutic decisions that support children's participation and engagement in play.

References

Accreditation Council for Occupational Therapy Education (ACOTE) Standards and Interpretive Guidelines. (2008). Retrieved April 15, 2009, from http://www.aota.org/Educate/Accredit/StandardsReview/guide/42369.aspx

Adams, B., Wilgosh, L., & Sobsey, D. (1990). Sorrow or commitment: The experience of being the parent of a child with severe disabilities. *Developmental Disabilities Bulletin, 18*(1), 49–58.

Aldis, O. (1975). *Play fighting.* New York: Academic Press.

Allard, H. (1985). *Miss Nelson is missing!* New York: Houghton Mifflin.

Allard, H. (1988). *Miss Nelson has a field day.* New York: Houghton Mifflin.

American Academy of Pediatrics. (2001). Committee on Public Education: Children, adolescents, and television. Policy statement. *Pediatrics, 107*, 423–426.

American Medical Association. (1943). Essentials of an acceptable school of occupational therapy. *Journal of the American Medical Association, 122*, 541–542.

American Occupational Therapy Association. (1975). Essentials of an accredited educational program for the occupational therapist. *American Journal of Occupational Therapy, 29*, 485–496.

American Occupational Therapy Association. (1993). Position paper: Purposeful activity. *American Journal of Occupational Therapy, 47*, 1081–1082.

American Occupational Therapy Association. (2007). *Societal statement on play.* Bethesda, MD: Americal Occupational Therapy Association..

American Occupational Therapy Association. (2008). Occupational therapy practice framework: Domain & process. *American Journal of Occupational Therapy, 62*, 625–683.

Anderson, J., & Hinojosa, J. (1984). Parents and therapists in a professional partnership. *American Journal of Occupational Therapy, 38*, 452–461.

Antle, B. J. (2004). Factors associated with self worth in young people with physical disabilities. *Health & Social Work, 29*, 167–175.

Apter, M. J. (1991). A structural-phenomenology of play. In J. H. Kerr & M. J. Apter (Eds.), *Adult play: A reversal theory approach* (pp. 13–29). Amsterdam: Swets & Zeitlinger.

Awaad, T. (2003). Culture, cultural competency, and occupational therapy: A review of the literature. *British Journal of Occupational Therapy, 66*, 356–362.

Ayres, A. J. (1963). The development of perceptual-motor abilities: A theoretical basis for treatment of dysfunction. *American Journal of Occupational Therapy, 17*, 221–225.

Ayres, A. J. (1964). Tactile functions: The relation to hyperactive and perceptual motor behavior. *Perceptual and Motor Skills, 20*, 288–292.

Ayres A. J. (1971). Characteristics of types of sensory integrative dysfunction. *American Journal of Occupational Therapy, 25*, 329–334.

Ayres, A .J. (1972). *Sensory integration and learning disorders.* Los Angeles: Western Psychological Services.

Ayres, A. J. (1979). *Sensory integration and the child.* Los Angeles: Western Psychological Services.

Ayres, A. J. (2005). *Sensory integration and the child: 25th anniversary edition.* Los Angeles: Western Psychological Services.

Baker, M. J., Koegel, R. L., & Koegel, L. K. (1998). Increasing the social behavior of young children with autism using their obsessive behaviors. *Journal of the Association for Persons with Severe Handicaps, 23*, 300–308.

Baranek, G. T., Reinhartsen, D. B., & Wannamaker, S. W. (2001). Play: Engaging young children with autism. In R. A. Huebner (Ed.), *Autism: A sensorimotor approach to management* (pp. 313–351). Gaithersburg, MD: Aspen.

Barnes, D. R. (2006). Play in historical and cross-cultural contexts. In D. P. Fromberg & D. Bergen (Eds.), *Play from birth to twelve.* (pp. 243–260). New York: Routledge.

Barnes, R. M. (1949). *Motion and time study* (3rd ed.). New York: John Wiley & Sons.

Barnett, L. A. (1990). Playfulness: Definition, design, and measurement. *Play and culture, 3*, 319–336.

Barnett, L. A. (1991). Characterizing playfulness: Correlates with individual attributes and personality traits. *Play & culture, 4*, 371–393.

Barnett, L. A. (2007). The nature of playfulness in young adults. *Personality and Individual Differences, 43*, 949–958.

Baron, K. B. (1991). The use of play in child psychiatry: Reframing the therapeutic environment. *Occupational Therapy in Mental Health, 11*(2/3), 37–56.

Barry, L. M., & Burlew, S. B. (2004). Using social stories to teach choice and play skills to children with autism. *Focus on Autism and Other Developmental Disabilities, 19*(1), 45–51.

Bateson, G. (1972). *Steps to an ecology of mind.* New York: Ballantine.

Bateson, P. (2005). The role of play in the evolution of great apes and humans. In A. D. Pellegrini & P. K. Smith (Eds.), *The nature of play: Great apes and humans* (pp. 13–24). New York: Guilford Press.

Bay-Hinitz, A. K., & Wilson, G. R. (2005). A cooperative games intervention for aggressive preschool children. In L. A. Reddy, T. M. Files-Hall, & C. E. Schaefer (Eds.), *Empirically based play interventions for children* (pp. 191–211). Washington, DC: American Psychological Association.

Bazyk, S., Stalnaker, D., Llerena, M., Ekelman, B., & Bazyk, J. (2003). Play in Mayan children. *American Journal of Occupational Therapy, 57,* 273–283.

Bekoff, M. (2002). *Minding animals.* London: Oxford University Press.

Bekoff, M., & Byers, J. A. (1998). *Animal play: Evolutionary, comparative, and ecological perspectives.* New York: Cambridge University Press.

Bell, A. C., & Dyment, J. E. (2006). Grounds for action: Promoting physical activity through school ground greening in Canada. Toyota Evergreen Learning Grounds Program. Retrieved September 19, 2008, from http://www.evergreen.ca/en/lg/pdf/PHACreport.pdf

Belsky, J., Goode, M. K., & Most, R. K. (1980). Maternal stimulation and infant exploratory competence: Cross-sectional, correlational, and experimental analyses. *Child Development, 51,* 1168–1178.

Belsky, J., & Most, R. K. (1981). From exploration to play: A cross sectional study of infant-free play behavior. *Developmental Psychology, 17,* 630–639.

Benenson, J. F. (1993). Greater preference among females than males for dyadic interaction in early childhood. *Child Development, 64,* 544–555.

Benjamin, H. (1932). Age and sex differences in toy preferences of young children. *Journal of Genetic Psychology, 41,* 417–429.

Benson, J. D., Nicka, M. N., & Stern, P. (2006). How does a child with sensory processing problems play? *Internet Journal of Allied Health Sciences and Practice, 4.* Retrieved July 28, 2008, from http://ijahsp.nova.edu/articles/vol4num4/benson.pdf

Berlyne, D. E. (1960). *Conflict, arousal, and curiosity.* New York: McGraw-Hill.

Bernard-Opitz, V., Ing, S., & Kong, T. Y. (2004). Comparison of behavioural and natural play interventions for young children with autism. *Autism, 8,* 319–333.

Biben, M. (1998). Squirrel monkeys playfighting: Making the case for a cognitive training function in play. In M. Bekoff & J. A. Byers (Eds.), *Animal play: Evolutionary, comparative, and ecological perspectives* (pp. 161–182). New York: Cambridge University Press.

Blanche, E. (1992). Creativity in sensory integrative treatment. *Sensory Integration Special Interest Section Newsletter, 15*(1), 3–4.

Blanche, E. I. (2008). Play in children with cerebral palsy: Doing with—not doing to. In L. D. Parham & L. S. Fazio (Eds.), *Play in occupational therapy for children* (2nd ed., pp. 375–393). St. Louis, MO: Mosby Elsevier.

Blunden, P. (2001). The therapeutic use of play. In L. Lougher (Ed.), *Occupational therapy for child and adolescent mental health* (pp. 67–86). Edinburgh, Scotland: Churchill Livingstone.

Blurton Jones, N. G. (1978). An ethological study of some aspects of social behavior of children in nursery school. In D. Muller-Schwarze (Ed.), *Evolution of play behavior* (pp. 349–366). Stroudsburg, PA: Dowden, Hutchinson & Ross.

Boxill, N. A., & Beaty, A. L. (1990). Mother/child interaction among homeless women and their children in a public night shelter in Atlanta, Georgia. In N. A. Boxill (Ed.), *Homeless children: The watchers and the waiters* (pp. 49–64). Binghamton, NY: Haworth Press.

Bracegirdle, H. (1992). The use of play in occupational therapy for children: How the therapist can help. *British Journal of Occupational Therapy, 55,* 201–202.

Bradbard, M. R., & Parkman, S. A. (1983). Gender differences in preschool children's toy requests. *Journal of Genetic Psychology, 145,* 283–285.

Bratton, S., & Ray, D. (2000). What the research shows about play therapy. *International Journal of Play Therapy, 9,* 47–88.

Bratton, S. C., Ray, D., Rhine, T., & Jones, L. (2005). The efficacy of play therapy with children: A meta-analytic review of treatment outcomes. *Professional Psychology: Research and Practice, 36,* 376–390.

Brazelton, T. B., Koslowski, B., & Main, M. (1974). The origins of reciprocity: The early mother-infant interaction. In M. Lewis & L. A. Rosenblum (Eds.), *The effect of the infant on its caregiver* (pp. 49–76). New York: John Wiley & Sons.

Brazelton, T. B., & Tronick, E. (1980). Preverbal communication between mothers and infants. In D. R. Olson (Ed.), *The social foundations of language and thought* (pp. 299–315). New York: Norton.

Brown, A. M., Humphry, R., & Taylor, E. (1997). A model of the nature of family-therapist relationships: Implications for education. *American Journal of Occupational Therapy, 51,* 597–603.

Brown, M., Christensen, K., Schroer, L., Steffan, J., Carlson, A., Giraud, A., et al. (2008, April). Perceived indicators of engagement in children with autism spectrum disorders participating in sensory-based activities. Poster presented at the annual conference of the American Occupational Therapy Association, Long Beach, CA.

Brown, M., & Gordon, W. (1987). Impact of impairment on activity patterns of children. *Archives of Physical Medicine and Rehabilitation, 68,* 828–832.

Brown, S. (1998). Play as an organizing principal: Clinical evidence and personal observations. In M. Bekoff & J. A. Byers (Eds.), *Animal play* (pp. 243–259). New York: Cambridge University Press.

Bruner, J. S. (1982). The organization of action and the nature of adult-infant transaction. In M. Cranach & R. Harre (Eds.), *The analysis of action* (pp. 313–327). New York: Cambridge University Press.

Bryze, K. C. (2008). Narrative contributions to the play history. In L. D. Parham & L. S. Fazio (Eds.), *Play in occupational therapy for children* (2nd ed., pp. 43–54). St. Louis, MO: Mosby Elsevier.

Buckley, K., & Poole, S. (2004). Activity analysis. In J. Hinohosa & M. Blount (Eds.), *Texture of life* (pp. 69–114). Bethesda, MD: AOTA Press.

Bundy, A. (1992). Play: The most important occupation of children. *American Occupational Therapy Association's Sensory Integration Special Interest Section Newsletter, 15*(2), 1–2.

Bundy, A. C. (1989). A comparison of the play skills of normal boys and boys with sensory integrative dysfunction. *Occupational Therapy Journal of Research, 9,* 84–100.

Bundy, A. C. (1993). Assessment of play and leisure: delineation of the problem. *American Journal of Occupational Therapy, 47,* 217–222.

Bundy, A. C. (1997). Play and playfulness: What to look for. In L. D. Parham & L. S. Fazio (Eds.), *Play in occupational therapy for children* (pp. 52–66). St. Louis, MO: Mosby.

Bundy, A. C., Luckett, T., Naughton, G. A., Tranter, P. J., Wyver, S. R., Ragen, J., et al. (2008). Playful interaction: Occupational therapy for all children on the school playground. *American Journal of Occupational Therapy, 62*, 522–527.

Bundy, A. C., & Murray, E. A. (2002). Sensory integration: A. Jean Ayres' theory revisited. In A. C. Bundy, S. J. Lane, & E. A. Murray (Eds.), *Sensory integration: Theory and practice* (2nd ed.). Philadelphia: F. A. Davis.

Burghardt, G. M. (1984). On the origins of play. In P. K. Smith (Ed.), *Play in animals and humans* (pp. 5–41). New York: Basil Blackwell.

Burghardt, G. M. (1998). The evolutionary origins of play revisited: Lessons from turtles. In M. Bekoff & J. A. Byers (Eds.), *Animal play: Evolutionary, comparative, and ecological perspectives* (pp. 1–26). New York: Cambridge University Press.

Burghardt, G. M. (2005). *The genesis of animal play: Testing the limits.* Cambridge, MA: MIT Press.

Burke, J. P., Schaaf, R. C., & Hall, T. B. L. (2008). Family narratives and play assessment. In L. D. Parham & L. S. Fazio (Eds.), *Play in occupational therapy for children* (2nd ed., pp. 195–215). St. Louis, MO: Mosby Elsevier.

Butcher, J. (1991). Development of a playground skills test. *Perceptual & Motor Skills, 72*, 259–266.

Byers, J. A. (1998). Biological effects of locomotor play: Getting into shape or something more specific. In M. Bekoff & J. A. Byers (Eds.), *Animal play: Evolutionary, comparative, and ecological perspectives* (pp. 205–220). New York: Cambridge University Press.

Caiazzo, L., Sarra, A., Vechionne, M., Miller, E., & Miller Kuhaneck, H. (2008). A survey of children's play preferences: Further examination of the Dynamic Model for Play Choice. Unpublished master's thesis, Sacred Heart University, Fairfield, CT.

Caldera, Y. M., Huston, A. C., & O'Brien, M. (1989). Social interactions and play patterns of parents and toddlers with feminine, masculine, and neutral toys. *Child Development, 60*(1), 70–76.

Canadian Association of Occupational Therapists. (1996). Practice paper: Occupational therapy and children's play. *Canadian Journal of Occupational Therapy, 63*(2), Insert 1–9.

Carlson, M. (1996). The self-perpetuation of occupations. In R. Zemke & F. Clark (Eds.), *Occupational science: The evolving discipline* (pp. 143–157). Philadelphia: F. A. Davis.

Caro, T. M. (1994). *Cheetahs of the Serengeti plains: Group living in an asocial species.* Chicago: University of Chicago Press.

Case-Smith, J. (1997). Variables related to successful school-based practice. *Occupational Therapy Journal of Research, 17*, 133–153.

Case-Smith, J. (2000). Effects of occupational therapy services on fine motor and functional performance in preschool children. *American Journal of Occupational Therapy, 54*, 372–380.

Case-Smith, J., & Miller Kuhaneck, H. (2008). Play preferences of typically developing children and children with developmental delays between the ages of 3 and 7 years. *OTJR: Occupation, Participation and Health, 28*, 19–29.

Case-Smith, J., Richardson, P., & Schultz-Krohn, W. (2005). *An overview of occupational therapy for children.* St. Louis, MO: Mosby.

Chandler, B. (Ed.). (1997). *The essence of play: a child's occupation.* Bethesda, MD: American Occupational Therapy Association.

Cherng, R. J., Chen, J. J., & Su, F. C. (2001). Vestibular system in performance of standing balance of children and young adults under altered sensory conditions. *Perceptual Motor Skills, 92*, 1167–1179.

Chew, T. (1985). *The developmental progression of vestibular based playground play of preschool children.* Unpublished master's thesis, University of Southern California, Los Angeles.

Chiang, M., & Carlson, G. (2003). Occupational therapy in multicultural contexts: Issues and strategies. *British Journal of Occupational Therapy, 66*, 559–567.

Chiarello, L. A., Huntington, A., & Bundy, A. (2006). A comparison of motor behaviors, interaction, and playfulness during mother-child and father-child play with children with motor delay: Implications for early intervention practice. *Occupational & Physical Therapy in Pediatrics, 26*(1/2), 129–152.

Christakis, D. A., Ebel, B. E., Rivara, F. P., & Zimmerman, F. J. (2004). Television, video, and computer game usage in children under 11 years of age. *Journal of Pediatrics, 145*, 652–656.

Christensen, P., & Mikkelsen, M. R. (2008). Jumping off and being careful: Children's strategies of risk management in everyday life. *Sociology of Health & Illness, 30*(1), 112–130.

Clements, R. (2004). An investigation of the status of outdoor play. *Contemporary Issues in Early Childhood, 5*(1), 68–80.

Clifford, J. M., & Bundy, A. (1989). Play preference and play performance in normal boys and boys with sensory integrative dysfunction. *Occupational Therapy Journal of Research, 9*, 202–217.

Cohen, L. (2001). *Playful parenting.* New York: Ballantine.

Cole, D., & LaVoie, J. C. (1985). Fantasy play and related cognitive development in 2 to 6 year olds. *Developmental Psychology, 21*, 233–240.

Cole, M. B., & McLean, V. (2003). Therapeutic relationships re-defined. *Occupational Therapy in Mental Health, 19*(2), 33–56.

Colman, W. (1990). Evolving educational practices in occupational therapy: The war emergency courses, 1936–54. *American Journal of Occupational Therapy, 44*, 1028–1036.

Colman, W. (1992). Structuring education: Development of the first educational standards in occupational therapy, 1917–1930. *American Journal of Occupational Therapy, 46*, 653–660.

Common Sense Media. (2008). *Media + child and adolescent health: A systematic review.* Retrieved December 5, 2008, from http://www.commonsensemedia.org/sites/default/files/CSM_media+health_v2c%20110708.pdf

Connor, J. M., & Serbin, L. A. (1977). Behaviorally based masculine and feminine activity preferences scales for preschoolers: Correlates with other classroom behaviors and cognitive tests. *Child Development, 48*, 1411–1416.

Cook, D. G. (1996). The impact of having a child with autism. *Developmental Disabilities Special Interest Section Newsletter, 19*(2), 1–4.

Cook, S., Peterson, L., & DiLillo, D. (1999). Fear and exhilaration in response to risk: An extension of a model of injury risk in a real-world context. *Behavior Therapy, 30*(1), 5–15.

Corsaro, W. A., & Eder, D. (1990). Children's peer cultures. *Annual Review of Sociology, 16*, 197–220.

Cottrell, R. (1996). *Perspectives on purposeful activity: Foundation and future of occupational therapy.* Bethesda MD: AOTA Press.

Couch, K. J., Deitz, J. C., & Kanny, E. M. (1998). The role of play in pediatric occupational therapy. *American Journal of Occupational Therapy, 52*, 111–117.

Creighton, C. (1992). The origin and evolution of activity analysis. *American Journal of Occupational Therapy, 46*, 45–48.

Crepeau, E. B. (1991). Achieving intersubjective understanding: Examples from an occupational therapy treatment session. *American Journal of Occupational Therapy, 45*, 1016–1025.

Crepeau, E. B. (2003). Analyzing occupation and activity: A way of thinking about occupational performance. In E. B. Crepeau, E. S. Cohn, & B. B. Schell (Eds.), *Willard & Spackman's occupational therapy* (10th ed., pp. 189–202). Philadelphia: Lippincott, Williams & Wilkins.

Csikszentmihalyi, M. (1990). *Flow: The psychology of optimal experience.* New York: Harper & Row.

Cummings, H. M., & Vandewater, E. A. (2007). Relation of adolescent video game play to time spent in other activities. *Archives of Pediatric and Adolescent Medicine, 161*, 684–689.

Curtin, C. (2001). Eliciting children's voices in qualitative research. *American Journal of Occupational Therapy, 55*, 295–302.

Damast, A. M., Tamis-LeMonda, C. S., & Bornstein, M. H. (1996). Mother-child play: Sequential interactions and the relation between maternal beliefs and behaviors. *Child Development, 67*, 1752–1766.

Darragh, A. R., Sample, P. L., & Krieger, S. R. (2001). "Tears in my eyes 'cause somebody finally understood": Client perceptions of practitioners following brain injury. *American Journal of Occupational Therapy, 55*, 191–199.

Daunhauer, L. A., Coster, W. J., Tickle-Degnen, L., & Cermak, S. A. (2007). Effects of caregiver-child interactions on play occupations among young children institutionalized in Eastern Europe. *American Journal of Occupational Therapy, 61*, 429–440.

Davies, S. L., Glaser, D., & Kossoff, R. (2000). Children's sexual play and behavior in pre-school settings: Staff perceptions, reports, and responses. *Child Abuse & Neglect, 24*, 1329–1343.

Da Vanzo, J., & Omar Rahman, M. (1993). American families: Trends and correlates. *Population Index. 59*, 350–386.

De Barros, K. M. F. T., Fragosos, A. G. C., de Oliveira, A. L. B., Filho, J. E. C., & de Castro, R. M. (2003). Do environmental influences alter motor abilities acquisition? *Arquivos de Neuro-psiquiatria, 61*, 170–175.

DeGangi, G. A., Wietlisbach, S., Goodin, M., & Scheiner, N. (1993). A comparison of structured sensorimotor therapy and child-centered activity in the treatment of preschool children with sensorimotor problems. *American Journal of Occupational Therapy, 47*, 777–786.

Deitz, J. C., & Swinth, Y. (2008). Accessing play through assistive technology. In L. D. Parham & L. S. Fazio (Eds.), *Play in occupational therapy for children* (2nd ed., pp. 395–412). St. Louis, MO: Mosby Elsevier.

Desha, L., Ziviani, J., & Rodger, S. (2003). Play preferences and behavior of preschool children with autistic spectrum disorder in the clinical environment. *Physical and Occupational Therapy in Pediatrics, 23*(1), 21–42.

Devereaux, E. B. (1984). Occupational therapy's challenge: The caring relationship. *American Journal of Occupational Therapy, 38*, 791–798.

DiCarlo, C. F., & Reid, D. H. (2004). Increasing pretend toy play of toddlers with disabilities in an inclusive setting. *Journal of Applied Behavior Analysis, 37*, 197–207.

DiCarlo, C. F., Reid, D. H., & Stricklin, S. B. (2003). Increasing toy play among toddlers with multiple disabilities in an inclusive classroom: A more-to-less, child-directed intervention continuum. *Research in Developmental Disabilities, 24*, 195–209.

Dunbar, S. (2007). *Occupational therapy models for intervention with children and families.* Thorofare, NJ: Slack.

Dunkerley, E., Tickle-Degnen, L., & Coster, W. J. (1997). Therapist-child interaction in the middle minutes of sensory integration treatment. *American Journal of Occupational Therapy, 51*, 799–807.

Dunn, J., Wooding, C., & Hermann, J. (1977). Mothers' speech to young children: Variation in context. *Developmental Medicine & Child Neurology, 19*, 629–638.

Dunn, W. (2000). *Best practice occupational therapy in community service with children and families.* Thorofare, NJ: Slack.

Dunn, W., McClain, L. H., Brown, C., & Youngstrom, M. J. (1998). The ecology of human performance. In M. E. Neistadt & E. B. Crepeau (Eds.), *Willard & Spackman's occupational therapy* (9th ed., pp. 525–535). Philadelphia: Lippincott Williams & Wilkins.

Dunning, H. (1972). Environmental occupational therapy. *American Journal of Occupational Therapy, 26*, 292–298.

Dunton, W. R. (1954). History and development of occupational therapy. In H. S. Willard & C. S. Spackman (Eds.), *Principles of occupational therapy* (2nd ed., pp. 1–10). Philadelphia: J. B. Lippincott.

Durig, A. (1996). *Autism and the crisis of meaning.* Albany: State University of New York Press.

Edwards, C. P. (2005). Children's play in cross cultural perspective: A new look at the six culture study. In F. F. McMahon, D. E. Lytle, & B. Sutton-Smith (Eds.), *Play & culture studies Volume 6: Play: An interdisciplinary synthesis* (Vol. 6, pp. 81–96). Lanham, MD: University Press of America.

Elgas, P. M., Klein, E., Kantor, R., & Fernie, D. E. (1988). Play and the peer culture: Play styles and object use. *Journal of Research in Childhood Education, 3*, 142–153.

Elkind, D. (2001). *The hurried child: Growing up too fast, too soon* (3rd ed.). Cambridge, MA: Da Capo Press.

Engel-Yeger, B., Jarus, T., & Law, M. (2007). Impact of culture on children's community participation in Israel. *American Journal of Occupational Therapy, 61*, 421–428.

Erickson, E. (1950). *Childhood and society.* New York: W. W. Norton.

Esdaile, S. A. (1996). A play focused intervention involving mothers of pre-schoolers. *American Journal of Occupational Therapy, 50*, 113–123.

Esdaile, S., & Sanderson, A. (1987). Teaching parents toy making: A practical guide to early intervention. *British Journal of Occupational Therapy, 50*, 266–271.

Evans, I. M., & Meyer, L. H. (1999). Modifying adult interactional style as positive behavioural intervention for a child with Rett syndrome. *Journal of Intellectual & Developmental Disability, 24*, 191–205.

Fagan, R. (1984). Play and behavioral flexibility. In P. K. Smith (Ed.), *Play in animals and humans* (pp. 159–174). New York: Basil Blackwell.

Fall, M., Navelski, L. F., & Welch, K. K. (2002). Outcomes of a play intervention for children identified for special education services. *International Journal of Play Therapy, 11*, 91–106.

Fein, G. G. (1981). Pretend play in childhood and integrative review. *Child Development, 52*, 1095–1118.

Feldhusen, J. F., & Goh, B. E. (1995). Assessing and accessing creativity: An integrative review of theory, research and development. *Creativity Research Journal, 8*, 231–247.

Ferland, F. (1997). *Play, children with physical disabilities and occupational therapy.* Ottawa, Ontario, Canada: University of Ottawa Press.

Ferland, F. (2005). *The Ludic model: Play, children with physical disabilities and occupational therapy* (2nd ed.). Ottawa, Ontario: Canadian Association of Occupational Therapists.

Ferrara, C., & Hill, S.D. (1980). The responsiveness of autistic children to the predictability of social and nonsocial toys. *Journal of Autism and Developmental Disorders, 10,* 51–57.

Fewell, R. R. (1986). *Play assessment scale* (5th revision). Seattle: University of Washington.

Fidler, G. S., & Fidler, J. W. (1963). *Occupational therapy: A communication process in psychiatry.* New York: Macmillan.

Fidler, G. S., & Velde, B. P. (1999). *Activities: Reality and symbol.* Thorofare, NJ: Slack.

Fiese, B. H. (1990). Playful relationships: A contextual analysis of mother-toddler interaction and symbolic play. *Child Development, 61,* 1648–1656.

Findji, F. (1993). Attentional abilities and maternal scaffolding in the first year of life. *International Journal of Psychology, 28,* 681–692.

Fine, G. A., & Sandstrom, K. L. (1988). *Knowing children: Participant observation with minors.* Newbury Park, CA: Sage.

Finegan, J. K., Niccols, G. A., Zacher, J. E., & Hood, J. E. (1991). The play activity questionnaire: A parent report measure of children's play preferences. *Archives of Sexual Behavior, 20,* 393–408.

Fleming, M. H. (1994). Conditional reasoning: Creating meaningful experiences. In C. Mattingly & M. H. Fleming (Eds.), *Clinical reasoning: Forms of inquiry in a therapeutic practice* (pp. 197–235). Philadelphia: F. A. Davis.

Florey, L. (1971). An approach to play and play development. *The American Journal of Occupational Therapy, 25,* 275–280.

Florey, L. L., & Greene, S. (2008). Play in middle childhood. In L. D. Parham & L. S. Fazio (Eds.), *Play in occupational therapy for children* (2nd ed., pp. 279–299). St. Louis, MO: Mosby Elsevier.

Frank, G. (2000). *Venus on wheels.* Berkeley: University of California Press.

Frank, J. D. (1958). The therapeutic use of self. *American Journal of Occupational Therapy, 12,* 215–225.

Friedman, S., Thompson, M.A., Crawley, S., Criticos, A., Drake, D., Iacobbo, M., et al. (1976). Mutual visual regard during mother-infant play. *Perceptual and Motor Skills, 42,* 427–431.

Frost, J. L., Shin, D., & Jacobs, P. J. (1998). Physical environments and children's play. In O. N. Saracho & B. Spodek (Eds.), *Multiple perspectives on play in early childhood education* (pp. 255–294). Albany: State University of New York Press.

Fry, D. (2005). Rough and tumble social play in humans. In A. D. Pellegrini & P. K. Smith (Eds.), *The nature of play: Great apes and humans* (pp. 54–85). New York: Guilford Press.

Furby, L., & Wilke, M. (1982). Some characteristics of infants preferred toys. *Journal of Genetic Psychology, 140* (2d Half), 207–210.

Gahnstrom-Strandqvist, K., Tham, K., Josephsson, S., & Borell, L. (2000). Actions of competence in occupational therapy practice. *Scandinavian Journal of Occupational Therapy, 7,* 15–25.

Gallimore, R., Weisner, T. S., Kaufman, S. Z., & Bernheimer, L. P. (1989). The social construction of ecocultural niches: Family accommodation of developmentally delayed children. *American Journal on Mental Retardation, 94,* 216–230.

Garner, B. P., & Bergen, D. (2006). Play development from birth to age four. In D. P. Fromberg & D. Bergen (Eds.), *Play from birth to twelve: Contexts, perspectives and meanings* (2nd ed., pp. 3–12). New York: Routledge.

Geist, R. & Kielhofner, G. (1998). *The pediatric volitional questionnaire.* Chicago: University of Illinois, Model of Human Occupation Clearinghouse.

Gilbreth, F. B. (1904). Science in management for the one best way to do work. In H. F. Merrill (Ed.), *Classics in management,* (pp. 245–294.) New York: American Management Association.

Gilfoyle, E. M. (1980). Caring: A philosophy for practice. *American Journal of Occupational Therapy, 34,* 517–521.

Gillett, J. N., & LeBlanc, L. A. (2007). Parent-implemented natural language paradigm to increase language and play in children with autism. *Research in Autism Spectrum Disorders, 1,* 247–255.

Ginsburg, K. R., American Academy of Pediatrics Committee on Communications, and American Academy of Pediatrics Committee on Psychosocial Aspects of Child and Family Health. (2007). The importance of play in promoting healthy child development and maintaining strong parent-child bonds. *Pediatrics, 119,* 182–191.

Glassner, B. (1976). Kid society. *Urban Education, 11*(1), 5–22.

Gleave, G. M. (1954). Occupational therapy in children's hospitals and pediatric service. In H. S. Willard & C. S. Spackman (Eds.), *Principles of occupational therapy* (2nd ed., pp. 138–167). Philadelphia: J.B. Lippincott.

Glynn, M. A. (1994). Effects of work task cues and play task cues on information processing, judgment, and motivation. *Journal of Applied Psychology, 79,* 34–45.

Goetze, H. (1994). Processes in person-centered play therapy. In J. Hellendoorn, R. van der Kooij, & B. Sutton-Smith (Eds.), *Play and intervention* (pp. 63–76) Albany: State University of New York Press.

Goldman, B. D., & Buysse, V. (2007). Friendships in very young children. In O. N. Saracho & B. Spodek (Eds.), *Contemporary perspectives on socialization and social development in early childhood education* (pp. 165–192). Charlotte, NC: Information Age.

Goldstein, J. (1995). Aggressive toy play. In A. D. Pellegrini (Ed.), *The future of play theory* (pp. 127–147). Albany: State University of New York Press.

Gomes, J., & Martin-Andrade, B. (2005). Fantasy play in apes. In A. D. Pellegrini & P. K. Smith (Eds.), *The nature of play: Great apes and humans* (pp. 139–172). New York: Guilford Press.

Gooch, P., & Living, R. (2004). The therapeutic use of videogames within secure forensic settings: A review of the literature and application to practice. *British Journal of Occupational Therapy, 67,* 332–341.

Goode, D. A. (1980). The world of the congenitally deaf-blind. In J. Jacobs (Ed.), *Mental retardation: A phenomenological approach* (pp. 187–207). Springfield, IL: Charles C. Thomas.

Goode, D. (1994). *A world without words: The social construction of children born deaf and blind.* Philadelphia: Temple University Press.

Gordon, N. S., Burke, S., Akil, H., Watson, S. J., & Panksepp, J. (2003). Socially-induced brain "fertilization": Play promotes brain derived neurotrophic factor transcription in the amygdala and dorsolateral frontal cortex in juvenile rats. *Neuroscience Letters, 341,* 17–20.

Gordon, W. R., & Caltabiano, M. L. (1996, Winter). Urban-rural differences in adolescent self-esteem, leisure boredom, and sensation-seeking as predictors of leisure-time usage and satisfaction. *Adolescence.* Retrieved July 21, 2008, from http://findarticles.com/p/articles/mi_m2248/is_n124_v31/ai_19226145

Gosso, Y., Otta, E., DeLima, M., Morais, S. E., Ribeiro, F. J. L., & Bussab, V. S. R. (2005). Play in hunter-gatherer society. In A. D. Pellegrini & P. K. Smith (Eds.), *The nature of play: Great apes and humans* (pp. 213–253). New York: Guilford Press.

Gottlieb, B. W., Gottlieb, J., Berkell, D., & Levy, L. (1986). Sociometric status and solitary play of LD boys and girls. *Journal of Learning Disabilities, 19*, 619–622.

Gowen, J. W., Johnson-Martin, N., Goldman, B. D., & Hussey, B. (1992). Object play and exploration in children with and without disabilities: A longitudinal study. *American Journal on Mental Retardation, 97*, 21–38.

Grandin, T. (1995). *Thinking in pictures and other reports from my life with autism.* New York: Doubleday.

Grandin, T., & Scariano, M. M. (1986). *Emergence: Labeled autistic.* Novato, CA: Arean Press.

Graue, M. E., & Walsh, D. J. (1995). Children in context: Interpreting the here and now of children's lives. In J. A. Hatch (Ed.), *Qualitative research in early childhood settings* (pp. 135–154). Westport, CT: Praeger.

Greenspan, S. I., & Wieder, S. (1997). An integrated developmental approach to interventions for young children with severe difficulties in relating and communicating. *Zero to Three, 17*, 5–17.

Griffiths, M. (2005). Video games and health: Video gaming is safe for most players and can be useful in health care. *British Medical Journal, 331*, 122–123. Retrieved July 8, 2008, from http://www.bmj.com/cgi/reprint/331/7509/122

Groos, K. (1901). *The play of man.* New York: Appleton.

Guidetti, S., & Tham, K. (2002). Therapeutic strategies used by occupational therapists in self-care training: A qualitative study. *Occupational Therapy International, 9*, 257–276.

Guitard, P., Ferland, F., & Dutil, E. (2005). Toward a better understanding of playfulness in adults. *OTJR: Occupation, Participation and Health, 25*, 9–22.

Gunter B., & Furnham, A. (1998) *Children as consumers.* London: Routledge.

Haas, L. J. (1925). *Occupational therapy for the mentally and nervously ill.* Milwaukee, WI: Bruce.

Haight, W. L., & Miller, P. J. (1992). The development of everyday pretend play: A longitudinal study of mothers' participation. *Merrill-Palmer Quarterly, 38*, 331–349.

Hall, E. T. (1982). *The hidden dimension.* Garden City, NY: Doubleday. (Original work published 1966).

Hall, S. I. (1998). Object play by adult animals. In M. Bekoff & J. A. Byers (Eds.), *Animal play: Evolutionary, comparative, and ecological perspectives* (pp. 45–60). New York: Cambridge University Press.

Halliday, S., & Leslie, J. C. (1986). A longitudinal cross-sectional study of the development of mother-child interaction. *British Journal of Developmental Psychology, 4*, 211–222.

Halverson, C. F., & Waldrop, M. F. (1973). The relations of mechanically recorded activity level to varieties of preschool play behavior. *Child Development, 44*, 678–681.

Hamm, E. M. (2006). Playfulness and the environmental support of play in children with and without disabilities. *OTJR: Occupation, Participation, & Health, 26*, 88–96.

Hampton, V. R. (1999). *The Penn Interactive Peer Play Scale for kindergarten: Building essential linkages in early childhood assessment.* Dissertation, University of Pennsylvania, Philadelphia. Retrieved June 17, 2008, from http://repository.upenn.edu/dissertations/AAI9953540.

Hanley, G. P., Cammilleri, A. P., Tiger, J. H., & Ingvarsson, E. T. (2007). A method for describing preschoolers' activity preferences. *Journal of Applied Behavior Analysis, 40*, 603–618.

Hanzlik, J. R. (1989). The effect of intervention on the free-play experience for mothers and their infants with developmental delay and cerebral palsy. *Physical and Occupational Therapy in Pediatrics, 9*(2), 33–51.

Harkness, L., & Bundy, A. C. (2001). Playfulness and children with physical disabilities. *Occupational Therapy Journal of Research, 21*, 73–89.

Harrington, M., & Dawson, D. (1997). Recreation as empowerment for homeless people living in shelters. *Journal of Leisurability, 24*(1). Retrieved June 26, 2008, from http://lin.ca/resource-details/892

Hartup, W. W. (1983). Peer relations. In P. H. Mussen (Ed.), *Handbook of child psychology* (4th ed., pp. 103–196). New York: Wiley.

Hartup, W. W. (1996). The company they keep: Friendships and their developmental significance. *Child Development, 67*, 1–13.

Hasselkus, B. R., & Dickie, V. A. (1994). Doing occupational therapy: Dimensions of satisfaction and dissatisfaction. *American Journal of Occupational Therapy, 48*, 145–154.

Heah, T., Case, T., McGuire, B., & Law, M. (2007). Successful participation: The lived experience among children with disabilities. *Canadian Journal of Occupational Therapy, 74*(1), 38–47.

Heal, N. A., & Hanley, G. P. (2007). Evaluating preschool children's preferences for motivational systems during instruction. *Journal of Applied Behavioral Analysis, 40*, 249–261.

Heinrich, B., & Smolker, R. (1998). Play in common ravens. In M. Bekoff & J. A. Byers (Eds.), *Animal play: Evolutionary, comparative, and ecological perspectives* (pp. 27–44). New York: Cambridge University Press.

Hektner, J. M., & Csikszentmihalyi, M. (1996, April). A longitudinal exploration of flow and intrinsic motivation in adolescents. Paper presented at the annual meeting of the American Educational Research Association, New York, NY. Retrieved July 21, 2008, from http://eric.ed.gov/ERICDocs/data/ericdocs2sql/content_storage_01/0000019b/80/14/84/e3.pdf

Hellendoorn, J. (1994). Imaginative play training for severely retarded children. In J. Hellendoorn, R. van der Kooij, & B. Sutton-Smith (Eds.), *Play and intervention* (pp. 113–122). Albany: State University of New York Press.

Henig, R. M. (2008, February 17). Taking play seriously. *New York Times.* Retrieved July 28, 2008, from http://www.nytimes.com/2008/02/17/magazine/17play.html?pagewanted=1

Henricks, T. S. (1999). Play as ascending meaning: Implications of a general model of play. In S. Reifel (Ed.), *Play & culture studies Volume 2: Play contexts revisited* (pp. 257–277). Westport, CT: Ablex.

Henry, A. D. (2000). *Kid play profile.* San Antonio, TX: Therapy Skill Builders.

Henry, A. (2008). Assessment of play and leisure in children and adolescents. In L. D. Parham & L. S. Fazio (Eds.), *Play in occupational therapy for children* (2nd ed., pp. 95–193). St. Louis, MO: Mosby Elsevier.

Hersch, G. I., Lamport, N. K., & Coffey, M. S. (2005). *Activity analysis: Application to occupation.* Thorofare, NJ: Slack.

Hinojosa, J. (2007). Becoming Innovators in an era of hyperchange (Eleanor Clarke Slagle Lecture). *American Journal of Occupational Therapy, 61*, 629–637.

Hinojosa, J., & Blount, M. (2004). Purposeful activities within the context of occupational therapy. In J. Hinojosa & M. Blount (Eds.), *Texture of life* (pp. 1–16). Bethesda, MD: AOTA Press.

Hinojosa, J., & Kramer, P. (2008). Integrating children with disabilities into family play. In L. D. Parham & L. S. Fazio (Eds.), *Play in occupational therapy for children* (2nd ed., pp. 321–334). St. Louis, MO: Mosby Elsevier.

Hoicka, E., & Gattis, M. (2008). Do the wrong thing: How toddlers tell a joke from a mistake. *Cognitive Development, 23*(1), 180–190.

Hol, T., Van den Berg, C. L., Van Ree, J. M., & Spruijt, B. M. (1999). Isolation during the play period in infancy decreases adult social interactions in rats. *Behavioral Brain Research, 100*, 91–97.

Holloway, E. (2008). Fostering early parent-infant playfulness in the neonatal intensive care unit. In L. D. Parham & L. S. Fazio (Eds.), *Play in occupational therapy for children* (2nd ed., pp. 335–350). St. Louis, MO: Mosby Elsevier.

Holmes, R. M. (1999). Kindergarten and college students' views of play and work at home and school. In S. Reifel (Ed.), *Play & culture studies Volume 2: Play contexts revisited.* (pp. 59–72). Stamford, CT: Ablex.

Honig, A. S. (2006). Sociocultural influences on gender role behaviors in children's play. In D. P. Fromberg & D. Bergen (Eds.), *Play from birth to twelve: Contexts, perspectives and meanings* (2nd ed., pp. 379–393). New York: Routledge.

Hoppes, S. (1997). Can play increase standing tolerance? A pilot-study. *Physical and Occupational Therapy in Geriatrics, 15*(1), 65–73.

Howard, A. C. (1986). Developmental play ages of physically abused and nonabused children. *American Journal of Occupational Therapy, 40*, 691–695.

Howard, J., Jenvey, V., & Hill, C. (2006). Children's categorization of play and learning based on social context. *Early Child Development and Care, 176*, 379–393.

Howard, L. (1996). A comparison of leisure time activities between able bodied children and children with physical disabilities. *British Journal of Occupational Therapy, 59*, 570–574.

Howle, J. (1997). *NDT in the United States: Changes in theory advance clinical practice.* Retrieved March 10, 2008, from http://www.paediatricworkshops.com.au/document/NDT_in_the_US.pdf

Howle J. (2002). *Neuro-developmental treatment approach: Theoretical foundations and principles of clinical practice.* Laguna Beach, CA: NDTA.

Huizinga, J. (1955). *Homo ludens: A study of the play-element in culture.* Boston: Beacon Press.

Humphreys, A., & Smith, P. K. (1987). Rough and tumble play, friendship and dominance in school children: Evidence for continuity and change with age. *Child Development, 58*, 201–212.

Humphry, R., & Wakeford, L. (2006). An occupation-centered discussion of development and implications for practice. *American Journal of Occupational Therapy, 60*, 258–267.

Hurff, J. M. (1981). Gaming technique: An assessment and training tool for individuals with learning deficits. *American Journal of Occupational Therapy, 35*, 728–735.

Hutt, C. (1966). Exploration and play in children. In P. A. Jewell & C. Loizos (Eds.), *Play, exploration and territory in mammals* (pp. 61–80). New York: Academic Press.

Ideishi, S. K., Ideishi, R. I., Gandhi, T., & Yuen, L. (2006, June). Inclusive preschool outdoor play environments. *School System Special Interest Section Quarterly, 13*(2), 1–4.

Incze, C. (n.d.). *Targeting skills based on a developmental play assessment: Effects of intervention on preschoolers with autism.* Master's thesis, Florida State University, Tallahassee. Retrieved July 23, 2008, from http://etd.lib.fsu.edu/theses/available/etd-07112005–110235/unrestricted/02_cci_text.pdf

Iwaniuk, A. N., Nelson, J. E., & Pellis, S. M. (2001). Do big brained animals play more? Comparative analyses of play and relative brain size in mammals. *Journal of Comparative Psychology, 115*, 29–41.

Jarrett, O. S., Farokhi, B., Young, C., & Davies, G. (2001). Boys and girls at play: Recess at a southern urban elementary school. In S. Reifel (Ed.), *Play & culture studies Volume 3: Theory in context and out* (pp. 147–170). Westport, CT: Ablex.

Johnson, J. E. (2006). Play development from ages four to eight. In D. P. Fromberg & D. Bergen (Eds.), *Play from birth to twelve: Contexts, perspectives and meanings* (2nd ed., pp. 13–20). New York: Routledge.

Johnson, J. E., Welteroth, S. J., & Corl, S. M. (2001). Attitudes of parents and teachers about play aggression in young children. In S. Reifel (Ed.), *Play & culture studies Volume 3: Theory in context and out* (pp. 335–354). Westport, CT: Ablex.

Kafai, Y. B. (1998). Video game designs by girls and boys: variability and consistency of gender differences. In J. Cassell & H. Jenkins (Eds.), *From Barbie to Mortal Kombat: Gender and computer games* (pp. 90–114). Cambridge, MA: MIT Press.

Kamei, N. (2005). Play among Baka children in Cameroon. In B. S. Hewlett & M. E. Lamb (Ed.), *Hunter-gatherer childhoods: Evolutionary, developmental & cultural perspectives* (pp. 343–362). New Brunswick, NJ: Transaction.

Kamitakahara, H., Monfils, M. H., Forgie, M. L., Kolb, B., & Pellis, S. M. (2007). The modulation of play fighting in rats: Role of the motor cortex. *Behavioral Neuroscience, 121*, 164–176.

Kantor, R., Elgas, P. M., & Fernie, D. E. (1993). Cultural knowledge and social competence within a preschool peer culture group. *Early Childhood Research Quarterly, 8*, 125–147.

Kaplan, E. B. (1997). *Not our kind of girl: Unraveling the myths of Black teenage motherhood.* Los Angeles: University of California.

Kaptchuk, T. J., Kelley, J. M., Conbody, L. A., Davis, R. B., Kerr, C. E., Jacobson, E. E., et al. (2008). Components of placebo effect: Randomized controlled trial in patients with irritable bowel syndrome. *British Medical Journal.* Retrieved June 9, 2008, from http://bmj.com/cgi/content/full/bmj.39524.439618.25v1

Kasari, C., Freeman, S., & Paparella, T. (2006). Joint attention and symbolic play in young children with autism: A randomized controlled intervention study. *Journal of Child Psychology & Psychiatry, 47*, 611–620.

Kearney, P. (2004). *The influence of competing paradigms on occupational therapy education: A brief history.* Retrieved June 27, 2007, from http://www.newfoundations.com/History/OccTher.html

Kelly-Byrne, D. (1989). *A child's play life: An ethnographic study.* New York: Teachers College.

Kibele, A. (2008, April). *Meaning in action: Toys and other objects in early childhood.* Presentation at the annual conference of the American Occupational Therapy Association, Long Beach, CA.

Kielhofner, G., & Barris, R. (1984). Collecting data on play: A critique of available methods. *Occupational Therapy Journal of Research, 4*, 150–180.

Kielhofner, G., Barris, R., Bauer, D., Shoestock, B., & Walker, L. (1983). A comparison of play behavior in nonhospitalized and hospitalized children. *American Journal of Occupational Therapy, 37*, 305–312.

Kim, Y. T., Lombardino, L. J., Rothman, H., & Vinson, B. (1989). Effects of symbolic play intervention with children who have mental retardation. *Mental Retardation, 27*, 159–165.

Kimball, J. (1999). Sensory integration frame of reference: Postulates regarding change and application to practice. In P. Kramer & J. Hinojosa (Eds.), *Frames of reference for pediatric cccupational therapy* (pp. 169–204). Baltimore: Lippincott Williams & Wilkins.

King, G., Law, M., King, S., Hurley, P., Hanna, S., Kertoy, M., et al. (2004). *Children's Assessment of Participation and Enjoyment (CAPE) and Preferences for Activities of Children (PAC)*. San Antonio, TX: Harcourt Assessment.

Kluth, P., & Schwarz, P. (2008). *"Just give him the whale!": 20 ways to use fascinations, areas of expertise, and strengths to support students with autism*. Baltimore: Paul H. Brookes.

Knox, S. (1974). A play scale. In M. Reilly (Ed.), *Play as exploratory learning* (pp. 247–266). Los Angeles: Sage.

Knox, S. H. (1993). Play and leisure. In H. L. Hopkins & H. D. Smith (Eds.), *Willard and Spackman's occupational therapy* (8th ed., pp. 260–268). Philadelphia: Lippincott.

Knox, S. H. (1997). *Play and play styles of preschool children*. Unpublished doctoral dissertation, University of Southern California, Los Angeles.

Knox, S. (2008). Development and current use of the revised Knox Preschool Play Scale. In L. D. Parham & L. S. Fazio (Eds.), *Play in occupational therapy for children* (2nd ed., pp. 55–70). St. Louis, MO: Mosby Elsevier.

Koegel, R. L., Dyer, K., & Bell, L. K. (1987). The influence of child-preferred activities on autistic children's social behavior. *Journal of Applied Behavior Analysis, 20*, 243–252.

Kohl, F. L., & Beckman, P. J. (1990). The effects of directed play on the frequency and length of reciprocal interactions with preschoolers having moderate handicaps. *Education & Training in Mental Retardation, 25*, 258–266.

Kok, A. J., Kong, T. Y., & Bernard-Opitz, V. (2002). A comparison of the effects of structured play and facilitated play approaches on preschoolers with autism: A case study. *Autism, 6*, 181–196.

Kraeger, M. M., & Walker, K. F. (1993). Attrition, burnout, job dissatisfaction and occupational therapy managers. *Occupational Therapy in Health Care, 8*, 47–62.

Kramer, P., & Hinojosa, J. (1999). *Frames of reference for pediatric occupational therapy*. Baltimore: Williams & Wilkins.

Lai, C. H., & Chan, Y. S. (2002). Development of the vestibular system. *Neuroembryology, 1*, 61–71.

Lally, J. R., & Stewart, J. (1990). *A guide to setting up environments: Infant/toddler caregiving*. Retrieved February 5, 2008, from California Department of Education, Center for Child and Family Studies Web site: http://clas.uiuc.edu/fulltext/cl03267/cl03267.html#pubinfo

Lancy, D. F. (1996). *Playing on the mother-ground: Cultural routines for children's development*. New York: Guilford Press.

Lane, S. J., & Mistrett, S. (2008). Facilitating play in early intervention. In L. D. Parham & L. S. Fazio (Eds.), *Play in occupational therapy for children* (2nd ed., pp. 413–425). St. Louis, MO: Mosby Elsevier.

Larsson, I., & Svedin, C. G. (2002). Teachers' and parents' reports on 3- to 6-year-old children's sexual behavior—A comparison. *Child Abuse & Neglect, 26*, 247–266.

Law, M. (1998). Does client-centered practice make a difference? In M. Law (Ed.), *Client-centered occupational therapy* (pp. 19–27). Thorofare, NJ: Slack.

Law, M., Missiuna, C., Pollock, N., & Stewart, D. (2005). Foundations for occupational therapy practice with children. In J. Case-Smith (Ed.), *Occupational therapy for children* (pp. 53–87). St. Louis, MO: Mosby.

Law, M., Polatajko, H., Baptiste, W., & Townsend, E. (1997). Core concepts of occupational therapy. In E. Townsend (Ed.), *Enabling occupation: An occupational therapy perspective* (pp. 29–56). Ottawa, Ontario, Canada: Canadian Association of Occupational Therapists.

Lawlor, M. C., & Mattingly, C. F. (1998). The complexities embedded in family-centered care. *American Journal of Occupational Therapy, 52*, 259–267.

Lawson, K. R., Parrinello, R., & Ruff, H. A. (1992). Maternal behavior and infant attention. *Infant Behavior and Development, 15*, 209–229.

Leipold, E., & Bundy, A. C. (2000). Playfulness and children with ADHD. *Occupational Therapy Journal of Research, 20*, 61–79.

Leister, C. A., Langenbrunner, M., & Walker, D. (1995). Pretend play: Opportunities to teach social interaction skills to young children with developmental disabilities. *Australian Journal of Early Childhood, 20*, 30–33.

Letts, L., Rigby, P., & Steward, D. (Eds.). (2003). *Using environments to enable occupational performance*. Thorofare, NJ: Slack.

Levin, D., & Rosenquest, B. (2001). The increase role of electronic toys in the lives of infants and toddlers: Should we be concerned? *Contemporary Issues in Early Childhood, 2*, 241–246.

Lewis, K. P. (2005). Social play in the great apes. In A. D. Pellegrini & P. K. Smith (Eds.), *The nature of play: Great apes and humans* (pp. 27–53). New York: Guilford Press.

Licht, S. (1967). The founding and the founders of the American Occupational Therapy Association. *American Journal of Occupational Therapy, 21*, 269–278.

Lieberman, J. N. (1965). Playfulness and divergent thinking: Investigation of their relationship at the kindergarten level. *Journal of Genetic Psychology, 107*, 219–224.

Lieberman, J. N. (1966). Playfulness: An attempt to conceptualize a quality of play and of the player. *Psychological Reports, 19*, 1278.

Lifter, K. (2000). Linking assessment to intervention for children with developmental disabilities or at-risk for developmental delay: The developmental play assessment (DPA) instrument. In K. Gitlin-Weiner, A. Sandgrund, & C. Schafer (Eds.), *Play diagnosis and assessment* (2nd ed., pp 228–261). New York: John Wiley & Sons.

Lifter, K., Ellis, J., Cannon, B., & Anderson, S. R. (2005). Developmental specificity in targeting and teaching play activities to children with pervasive developmental disorders. *Journal of Early Intervention, 27*, 247–267.

Linder, T. W. (1993). *Transdisciplinary play-based assessment: A functional approach to working with young children* (2nd ed.). Baltimore: Paul H. Brookes Publishing Company.

Linder, T. (2000). Transdisciplinary play-based assessment. In K. Gitlin-Weiner, A. Sandgrund, & C. Schafer (Eds.), *Play diagnosis and assessment* (2nd ed., pp 139–166). New York: John Wiley & Sons.

Livesay, H. (2007). Making a place for the angry hero on the team. In R. C. Lawrence (Ed.), *Using superheroes in counseling and play therapy* (pp. 121–142). New York: Springer.

Llorens, L. A. (1973). Activity analysis for cognitive-perceptual-motor dysfunction. *American Journal of Occupational Therapy, 27*, 453–456.

Llorens, L. A. (1986). Activity analysis: Agreement among factors in a sensory processing model. *American Journal of Occupational Therapy, 40,* 103–110.

Llorens, L. A. (1993). Activity analysis: Agreement between participants and observers on perceived factors in occupation components. *Occupational Therapy Journal of Research, 13,* 198–211.

Lloyd, C., & Maas, F. (1991). The therapeutic relationship. *British Journal of Occupational Therapy, 54,* 111–113.

Lowe, M. (1975). Trends in the development of representational play in infants from one to three years—an observational study. *Journal of Child Psychology and Psychiatry, 16*(1), 33–47.

Luecke, (2004). The history of pediatrics at Baylor University Medical Center. *Proceedings of the Baylor University Medical Center, 17,* 56–60. Retrieved August 15, 2008, from http://www.pubmedcentral.nih.gov/articlerender.fcgi?artid=1200641

Lyytinen, P., Laakso, M. L., Poikkeus, A. M., & Rita, N. (1999). The development and predictive relations of play and language across the second year. *Scandinavian Journal of Psychology, 40,* 177–186.

Malone, D. M., & Langone, J. (1999). Teaching object-related play skills to preschool children with developmental concerns. *International Journal of Disability, Development and Education, 46,* 325–336.

Manning, M. L. (2006). Play development from ages eight to twelve. In D. P. Fromberg & D. Bergen (Eds.), *Play from birth to twelve: Contexts, perspectives and meanings* (2nd ed., pp. 21–30). New York: Routledge.

Martin, C. L., Eisenbud, L., & Rose, H. (1995). Children's gender-based reasoning about toys. *Child Development, 66,* 1453–1471.

Martin, C. L., & Little, J. K. (1990). The relation of gender understanding to children's sex-typed preferences and gender stereotypes. *Child Development, 61,* 1427–1439.

Mastrangelo, S. (2009). Play and the child with autism spectrum disorder: From possibilities to practice. *International Journal of Play Therapy, 18*(1), 13–30.

Maternal and Child Health Bureau. (2005). *Family-centered care fact sheet.* Retrieved July 8, 2008, from http://www.medicalhomeinfo.org/publications/family.html

Matheson, C., Olsen, R. J., & Weisner, T. (2007). A good friend is hard to find: Friendship among adolescents with disabilities. *American Journal of Mental Retardation, 112,* 319–329.

Mattingly, C. (2006). Pocahontas goes to the clinic: Popular culture as Lingua Franca in a cultural borderland. *American Anthropologist, 108,* 494–501.

Mattingly, C., & Fleming, M. H. (1994). Interactive reasoning: Collaborating with the person. In C. Mattingly & M. H. Fleming (Eds.), *Clinical reasoning: Forms of inquiry in a therapeutic practice* (pp. 178–196). Philadelphia: F. A. Davis.

Mayeroff, M. (1971). *On caring.* New York: Harper Perennial.

McColl, M. A. (2003). Spirituality and disability. In M. A. McColl (Ed.), *Spirituality and occupational therapy* (pp. 19–30). Ottawa, Ontario, Canada: Canadian Association of Occupational Therapists.

McConkey, R. (1994). Families at play: Interventions for children with developmental handicaps. In J. Hellendoorn, R. van der Kooij, & B. Sutton-Smith (Eds.), *Play and intervention* (pp. 123–132). Albany: State University of New York Press.

McDaniel, M. L. (n.d.) *Occupational therapists before World War II (1917–40).* Retrieved July, 18, 2007, from http://history.amedd.army.mil/booksdocs/histories/ArmyMedicalSpecialistCorps/chapter4.htm#f

McEwen, M. (1990). The human-environment interface in occupational therapy: A theoretical and philosophical overview. In S. C. Merrill (Ed.), *Environment: Implications for occupational therapy practice, a sensory integrative perspective* (pp. 3–20). Rockville, MD: American Occupational Therapy Association.

McGhee, P. E. (1984). Play, incongruity and humor. In T. D. Yawkey & A. D. Pelligrini (Eds.), *Child's play: Developmental and applied.* (pp. 219–236). Hillsdale, NJ: Lawrence Erlbaum Associates.

McNary, H. (1954). The scope of occupational therapy. In H. S. Willard & C. S. Spackman (Eds.), *Principles of occupational therapy* (2nd ed., pp. 11–23). Philadelphia: J. B. Lippincott.

Media Analysis Laboratory. (1998). *Video game culture: Leisure and play preferences of B.C. teens.* Media Awareness Network. Retrieved October 20, 2005, from http://www.media-awareness.ca/english/resources/research_documents/studies/video_games/video_game_culture.cfm

Messer, D. J., & Vietze, P. M. (1984). Timing and transitions in mother-infant gaze. *Infant Behavior and Development, 7,* 167–181.

Messier, J., Ferland, F., & Majnemer, A. (2008). Play behavior of school age children with intellectual disability: Their capacities, interests and attitude. *Journal of Developmental and Physical Disabilities, 20,* 193–207.

Meyer, A. (1922). The philosophy of occupational therapy. *Archives of Occupational Therapy, 1,* 1–10.

Meyer-Bahlburg, H. F., Sandberg, D. E., Dolezal, C. L., & Yager, T. J. (1994). Gender-related assessment of childhood play. *Journal of Abnormal Child Psychology, 22,* 643–60.

Millar, S. (1968). *The psychology of play.* Baltimore: Penguin.

Miller, E., & Kuhaneck, H. (2008). Children's perceptions of play experiences and play preferences: A qualitative study. *American Journal of Occupational Therapy, 62,* 407–415.

Miller, E., & Miller-Kuhaneck, H. (2008, April). *Application of the dynamic model for play choice.* Paper presented at the annual conference of the American Occupational Therapy Association, Long Beach, CA.

Miller, H. (1996). Eye contact and gaze aversion: Implications for persons with autism. *Sensory Integration Special Interest Section Newsletter, 19*(2), 1–3.

Missiuna, C., & Pollack, N., (1991). Play deprivation in children with physical disabilities: The role of the occupational therapist preventing secondary disability. *American Journal of Occupational Therapy, 45,* 882–888.

Missiuna, C., Pollock, N., & Law, M. (2004). *The perceived efficacy and goal setting system.* San Antonio, TX: PsychCorp.

Mogford-Bevan, K. (2000). The Play Observation Kit (POKIT): An observational assessment technique for young children. In K. Gitlin-Weiner, A. Sandgrund, & C. Schafer (Eds.), *Play diagnosis and assessment* (2nd ed., pp. 262–302). New York: John Wiley & Sons.

Mook, B. (1994). Therapeutic play: From interpretation to intervention. In J. Hellendoorn, R. van der Kooij, & B. Sutton-Smith (Eds.), *Play and intervention* (pp. 39–52). Albany: State University of New York Press.

Moor, J. (2002). *Playing, laughing and learning with children on the autism spectrum: A practical resource of play ideas for parents and carers.* Philadelphia: Jessica Kingsley.

Moore, M., & Russ, S. W. (2006). Pretend play as a resource for children: Implications for pediatricians and health professionals. *Journal of Developmental & Behavioral Pediatrics, 27,* 237–248.

Morrongiello, B. A., & Lasenby-Lessard, J. (2007). Psychological determinants of risk-taking by children: An integrative model and implications for interventions. *Injury Prevention, 13,* 20–25.

Morrongiello, B. A., & Matheis, S. (2007a). Addressing the issue of falls off playground equipment: An empirically-based intervention to reduce fall-risk behavior on playgrounds. *Journal of Pediatric Psychology, 32,* 819–830.

Morrongiello, B. A., & Matheis, S. (2007b). Understanding children's injury-risk behaviors: The independent contributions of cognitions and emotions. *Journal of Pediatric Psychology, 32*(8), 926–937.

Mosey, A. C. (1981). *Occupational therapy: Configuration of a profession.* New York: Raven Press.

Mosey, A. C. (1986). *Psychosocial components of occupational therapy.* New York: Raven Press.

Moszkowski, R. J., & Stack, D. M. (2007). Infant touching behaviour during mother-infant face-to-face interactions. *Infant and Child Development, 16,* 307–319.

Mulderji, K. J. (1997). Peer relations and friendships in physically disabled children. *Child Care, Health & Development, 23,* 379–389.

Munier, V., Myers, C. T., & Pierce, D. (2008). Power of object play for infants and toddlers. In L. D. Parham & L. S. Fazio (Eds.), *Play in occupational therapy for children* (2nd ed., pp. 219–249). St. Louis, MO: Mosby Elsevier.

Munoz, J. P. (2007). Culturally responsive caring in occupational therapy. *Occupational Therapy International, 14,* 256–280.

Murphy, J. (2005). A haven for child's play. *Save the Children.* Retrieved June 26, 2008, from http://www.savethechildren.org/newsroom/2005/a-haven-for-childs-play.html

Muys, V., Rodger, S., & Bundy, A. C. (2006). Assessment of playfulness in children with autistic disorder: A comparison of the Children's Playfulness Scale and the Test of Playfulness. *OTJR: Occupation, Participation, & Health, 26,* 159–170.

Nadel, J., Martini, M., Field, T., Escalona, A., & Lundy, B. (2008). Children with autism approach more imitative and playful adults. *Early Child Development and Care, 178,* 461–465.

Nadworny, M. J. (1957). Frederick Taylor and Frank Gilbreth: Competition in scientific management. *Business History Review, 31,* 23–34.

Neistadt, M. E., McAuley, D., Zecha, D., & Shannon, R. (1993). An analysis of a board game as a treatment activity. *American Journal of Occupational Therapy, 47,* 154–160.

Nelson, D. L. (1996). Therapeutic occupation: A definition. *American Journal of Occupational Therapy, 50,* 775–782.

Nelson, J. K. (2008). Laugh and the world laughs with you: An attachment perspective on the meaning of laughter in psychotherapy. *Clinical Social Work Journal, 36*(1), 41–49.

Nevile, M., & Bachor, D. G. (2002). A script-based symbolic play intervention for children with developmental delay. *Developmental Disabilities Bulletin, 30,* 140–172.

Nilsen, D. L. F., & Nilsen, A. P. (1978). *Language play: An introduction to linguistics.* Rowley, MA: Newbury House.

Noll, L. M., & Harding, C. G. (2003). The relationship of mother-child interaction and the child's development of symbolic play. *Infant Mental Health Journal, 24,* 557–570.

Nwokah, E. E., & Ikekeonwu, C. (1998). A sociocultural comparison of Nigerian and American children's games. In M. C. Duncan, G. Chick, & A. Aycock (Eds.), *Play & culture studies Volume 1: Diversions and divergences in fields of play* (pp. 59–76). Greenwich, CT: Ablex.

O'Brien, J., Boatwright, T., Chaplin, J., Geckler, C., Gosnell, D., Holcombe, J., et al. (1998). The impact of positioning equipment on play skills of physically impaired children. In M. Carlisle Duncan, G. Chick, & A. Aycock (Eds.), *Play & culture studies Volume 1: Diversions and divergences in fields of play.* (pp. 149–160). Greenwich, CT: Ablex.

O'Brien, J., Coker, P., Lynne, R., Suppinger, R., Pearigen, T., Rabon, S., et al. (2000). The impact of occupational therapy on a child's playfulness. *Occupational Therapy in Health Care, 12*(2/3), 39–51.

O'Brien, M., & Huston, A. C. (1985). Activity level and sex-stereotyped toy choice in toddler boys and girls. *Journal of Genetic Psychology, 146,* 527–533.

Okimoto, A. M., Bundy, A., & Hanzlik, J. (2000). Playfulness in children with and without disability: Measurement and intervention. *American Journal of Occupational Therapy, 54,* 73–82.

Olson, L., Heaney, C., & Soppas-Hoffman, B. (1989). Parent-child activity group treatment in preventive psychiatry. *Occupational Therapy in Health Care, 6,* 29–43.

Paley, V. G. (1990). *The boy who would be a helicopter: The uses of storytelling in the classroom.* Cambridge, MA: Harvard University Press.

Palmadottir, G. (2003). Client perspectives on occupational therapy in rehabilitation services. *Scandinavian Journal of Occupational Therapy, 10,* 157–166.

Palmadottir, G. (2006). Client-therapist relationships: Experiences of occupational therapy clients in rehabilitation. *British Journal of Occupational Therapy, 69,* 394–401.

Panksepp, J., & Burgdorf, J. (2003). "Laughing" rats and the evolutionary antecedents of human joy? *Physiology & Behavior, 79,* 533–547.

Panksepp, J., Burgdorf, J., Turner, C., & Gordon, N. (2003). Modeling ADHD-type arousal with unilateral frontal cortex damage in rats and beneficial effects of play therapy. *Brain & Cognition, 52,* 97–105.

Parham, D. (1987). Nationally speaking—toward professionalism: The reflective therapist. *American Journal of Occupational Therapy, 41,* 555–561.

Parham, L. D. (1992). Strategies for maintaining a playful atmosphere during therapy. *Sensory Integration Special Interest Section Newsletter, 15*(1), 2–3.

Parham, L. D. (1996). Perspectives on play. In R. Zemke & F. Clark (Eds.), *Occupational science: The evolving discipline* (pp. 71–88). Philadelphia: F. A. Davis.

Parham, L. D. (2007). Play and occupational therapy. In L. D. Parham & L. S. Fazio (Eds.), *Play in occupational therapy for children* (2nd ed., pp. 3–42). St. Louis, MO: Mosby.

Parham, L. D., Cohn, E. S., Spitzer, S., Koomar, J. A., Miller, L. J., Burke, J. P., et al.(2007). Fidelity in sensory integration intervention research. *American Journal of Occupational Therapy, 61,* 216–227.

Parham, L. D., & Fazio, L. S. (1996). *Play in occupational therapy for children.* St. Louis, MO: Mosby.

Parham, L. D., & Fazio, L. S. (2007). *Play in occupational therapy for children* (2nd ed.). St. Louis, MO: Mosby.

Parham, L. D., & Mailloux, Z. (2005). Sensory integration. In J. Case-Smith (Ed.), *Occupational therapy for children.* St. Louis, MO: Mosby.

Parten, M. B. (1932). Social participation among preschool children. *Journal of Abnormal psychology, 27,* 243–69.

Pawelko, K. A., & Magafas, A. H. (1997, July). Leisure well being among adolescent groups: Time choices and self determination. *Parks & Recreation.* Retrieved July, 21, 2008, from http://findarticles.com/p/articles/mi_m1145/is_n7_v32/ai_19649715/pg_1?tag=artBody;col1

Pawlby, S. J. (1977). Imitative interaction. In H. R. Schaffer (Ed.), *Studies in mother-infant interaction* (pp. 203–224). London: Academic Press.

Pellegrini, A. D. (1988). Elementary-school children's rough-and-tumble play and social competence. *Developmental Psychology, 24,* 802–806.

Pellegrini, A. D. (1992). Preference for outdoor play during early adolescence. *Journal of Adolescence, 15,* 241–254.

Pellegrini, A. D. (1993). Boys' rough-and-tumble play, social competence, and group composition. *British Journal of Developmental Psychology, 11,* 237–248.

Pellegrini, A. D. (1994). The rough play of adolescent boys of differing sociometric status. *International Journal of Behavioral Development, 17,* 525–540.

Pellegrini, A. D. (1995). Boys' rough-and-tumble play and social competence. In A. D. Pellegrini (Ed.), *The future of play theory* (pp. 107–126). Albany: State University of New York Press.

Pellegrini, A. D. (2006). Rough and tumble play from childhood to adolescence. In D. P. Fromberg & D. Bergen (Eds.), *Play from birth to twelve: Contexts, perspectives and meanings* (2nd ed., pp. 111–118). New York: Routledge.

Pellegrini, A. D., & Bjorklund, D. E. (2004). The ontogeny and phylogeny of children's object and fantasy play. *Human Nature, 15,* 23–42.

Pellegrini, A. D., & Smith, P. K. (1998a). Physical activity play: The nature and function of a neglected aspect of play. *Child Development, 69,* 577–598.

Pellegrini, A. D., & Smith, P. K. (1998b). The development of play during childhood: Forms and possible function. *Child Psychology & Psychiatry Review, 3*(2), 51–57.

Pellegrini, A. D., & Smith, P. K. (2005). Play in the great apes and humans. In A. D. Pellegrini & P. K. Smith (Eds.), *The nature of play: Great apes and humans* (pp. 3–24). New York: Guilford Press.

Pellis, S. M., Hastings, E., Shimizu, T., Kamitakahara, H., Komorowska, J., Forgie, M. L., et al. (2006). The effects of orbital frontal cortex damage on the modulation of defensive responses by rats in playful and nonplayful social contexts. *Behavioral Neuroscience, 120*(1), 72–84.

Pellis, S. M., & Iwaniuk, A. N. (2002). Brain system size and adult-adult play in primates: A comparative analysis of the roles of the non-visual neocortex and the amygdala. *Behavioral Brain Research, 134,* 31–39.

Peloquin, S. M. (1990). The patient-therapist relationship in occupational therapy: Understanding visions and images. *American Journal of Occupational Therapy, 44,* 13–21.

Peloquin, S. M. (1993). The depersonalization of patients: A profile gleaned from narratives. *American Journal of Occupational Therapy, 47,* 830–837.

Peloquin, S. M. (1995). The fullness of empathy: Reflections and illustrations. *American Journal of Occupational Therapy, 49,* 24–31.

Petr, C. G., & Barney, D. D. (1993). Reasonable efforts for children with disabilities: The parents' perspective. *Social Work, 38,* 247–254.

Piaget, J. (1975). *The origins of intelligence in children.* New York: International Universities Press. (Original work published 1952).

Piaget, J. (1962). *Play, dreams and imitation in childhood.* New York: Norton.

Pierce, D. (2000). Maternal management of the home as a developmental play space for infants and toddlers. *American Journal of Occupational Therapy, 54,* 290–299.

Pluhar, E. (2007). Childhood sexuality. In M. S. Tepper & A. F. Owens (Eds.), *Sexual health, Volume 1: Psychological foundations* (pp. 155–181). Westport, CT: Praeger.

Polatajko, H. J., & Mandich, A. (2004). *Enabling occupation in children: The Cognitive Orientation to daily Occupational Performance (CO-OP) approach.* Ottawa, Ontario, Canada: CAOT Publications ACE.

Pollack, N., Stewart, D., Law, M., Sahagian-Whalen, S., Harvey, S., & Toal, C. (1997). The meaning of play for young people with physical disabilities. *Canadian Journal of Occupational Therapy, 64,* 25–31.

Porter, C., & Bundy, A. C. (2001). Validity of three tests of playfulness with African American children and their parents and relationships among parental beliefs and values and children's observed playfulness. In S. Reifel (Ed.), *Theory in context and out* (pp. 315–334). Westport, CT: Ablex.

Poulsen, A., & Ziviani, J. (2006). Children's participation beyond the school grounds. In S. Rodger & J. Ziviani (Eds.), *Occupational therapy with children: Understanding children's occupations and enabling participation* (pp. 280–298). Oxford, England: Blackwell.

Power, T. G. (2000). *Play and exploration in children and animals.* Mahwah, NJ: Lawrence Erlbaum.

Power, T. J., & Radcliffe, J. (2000). Assessing the cognitive ability of infants and toddlers through play: The symbolic play test. In K. Gitlin-Weiner, A. Sandgrund, & C. Schaefer (Eds.), *Play diagnosis and assessment* (2nd ed., pp. 58–79). New York: Wiley.

Price, P. (2009). The therapeutic relationship. In E. B. Crepeau, E. S. Cohn, & B. A. Boyt Schell (Eds.), *Willard & Spackman's occupational therapy* (11th ed., pp. 328–341). Philadelphia: Lippincott Williams & Wilkins.

Price, P., & Miner, S. (2007). Occupation emerges in the process of therapy. *American Journal of Occupational Therapy, 61,* 441–450.

Primeau, L. A. (1998). Orchestration of work and play within families. *American Journal of Occupational Therapy, 52,* 188–195.

Punwar, A. J. (2000). The art and science of practice. In A. J. Punwar & S. M. Peloquin (Eds.), *Occupational therapy principles and practice* (3rd ed., pp. 93–108). Philadelphia: Lippincott Williams & Wilkins.

Quilitch, H. R., & Risley, T. R. (1973). The effects of play materials on social play. *Journal of Applied Behavior Analysis, 6,* 573–578.

Raney, A. A., Smith, J. K., & Baker, K. (2006). Adolescents and the appeal of video games. In P. Vorderer & J. Bryant (Eds.), *Playing video games: Motives, responses, and consequences* (pp. 165–179). Mahwah, NJ: Erlbaum.

Reddy, L. A., Files-Hall, T. M., & Schaefer, C. E. (Eds.) (2005). *Empirically based play interventions for children.* Washington, DC: American Psychological Association.

Reed, C. N., Dunbar, S. B., & Bundy, A. C. (2000). The effects of an inclusive preschool experience on the playfulness of children with and without autism. *Physical and Occupational Therapy in Pediatrics, 19,* 73–89.

Reed, K. L., & Sanderson, S. (1999). *Concepts of occupational therapy.* Philadephia: Lippincott, Williams & Wilkins.

Reed, T. L. (2005). A qualitative approach to boys' rough and tumble play: There is more than meets the eye. In F. F. McMahon, D. E. Lytle, & B. Sutton-Smith (Eds.), *Play & culture studies Volume 6: Play: An interdisciplinary synthesis* (pp. 53–71). Lanham, MD: University Press of America.

Reid, D. (2004). The influence of virtual reality on playfulness in children with cerebral palsy: A pilot study. *Occupational Therapy International, 11*, 131–144.

Reid, D. H., DiCarlo, C. F., Schepis, M. M., Hawkins, J., & Stricklin, S. B., (2003). Observational assessment of toy preferences among young children with disabilities in inclusive settings: Efficiency analysis and comparison with staff opinion. *Behavior Modification, 27*, 233–250.

Reilly, M. (1974). Defining a cobweb. In M. Reilly (Ed.), *Play as exploratory learning: Studies of curiosity behavior* (pp. 57–116). London: Sage.

Reinhartsen, D. B., Garfinkle, A. N., & Wolery, M. (2002). Engagement with toys in two-year-old children with autism: Teacher selection versus child choice. *Research and Practice for Persons with Severe Disabilities, 27*, 175–187.

Renninger, K. A. (1990). Children's play interests, representation, and activity. In R. Fivush & J. A. Hudson (Eds.), *Knowing and remembering in young children* (pp. 127–165). New York: Cambridge University Press.

Restall, G., & Magill-Evans, J. (1994). Play and preschool children with autism. *American Journal of Occupational Therapy, 48*, 113–120.

Retting, M. (1994). The play of young children with visual impairments: Characteristics and interventions. *Journal of Visual Impairment & Blindness, 88*, 410–420.

Richmond, J. B. (1995). The Hull House era: Vintage years for children. *American Journal of Orthopsychiatry, 65*(1), 10–20.

Rigby, P., & Huggins, L. (2003). Enabling young children to play by creating supportive play environments. In L. Letts, P. Rigby, & D. Stewart (Eds.), *Using environments to enable occupational performance* (pp. 155–176). Thorofare, NJ: Slack.

Rigby, P., & Rodger, S. A. (2006). Developing as a player. In S. Rodger & J. Ziviani (Eds.), *Occupational therapy with children: Understanding children's occupations and enabling participation* (pp. 177–199). Oxford, England: Blackwell.

Rivkin, M. S. (2006). Children's outdoor play: An endangered activity. In D. P. Fromberg & D. Bergen (Eds.), *Play from birth to twelve: Contexts, perspectives and meanings* (2nd ed., pp. 323–330). New York: Routledge.

Roach M A., Barratt M S., Miller J F., & Leavitt L A. (1998). The structure of mother-child play: Young children with Down syndrome and typically developing children. *Developmental psychology, 34*(1), 77–87.

Roberts, M. C., Mitchell, M. C., & McNeal, R. (2003). The evolving field of pediatric psychology. In M. C. Roberts (Ed.), *Handbook of pediatric psychology* (pp. 3–18). New York: Guilford Press.

Rodger, S., & Ziviani, J. (Eds.) (2006). *Occupational therapy with children: Understanding children's occupations and enabling participation.* Oxford, England: Blackwell.

Rogers, C. S., Impara, J. C., Frary, R. B., Harris, T., Meeks, A., Semanic-Lauth, S., et al. (1998). Measuring playfulness: Development of the Child Behaviors Inventory of Playfulness. In M. C. Duncan, G. Chick, & A. Aycock (Eds.), *Play & culture studies Volume 1: Diversions and divergences in fields of play* (pp. 121–136). Greenwich, CT: Ablex.

Rogers, S. J. (2005). Play interventions for young children with autism spectrum disorders. In L. A. Reddy, T. M. Files-Hall, & C. E. Schaefer (Eds.), *Empirically based play interventions for children* (pp. 215–239). Washington, DC: American Psychological Association.

Rogers, S. J., Cook, I., & Meryl, A. (2005). Imitation and play in autism. In F. R. Volkmar, R. Paul, A. Klin, & D. J. Cohen, (Eds.), *Handbook of autism and pervasive developmental disorders, diagnosis, development, neurobiology and behavior.* (pp. 382–405). Hoboken, NJ: John Wiley & Sons.

Rosa, S. A., & Hasselkus, B. R. (1996). Connecting with patients: The personal experience of professional helping. *Occupational Therapy Journal of Research, 16*, 245–260.

Royeen, C. B., & Duncan, M. (1999). Acquisition frame of reference. In P. Kramer & J. Hinojosa (Eds.), *Frames of reference for pediatric occupational therapy* (pp. 377–400). Baltimore: Lippincott Williams & Wilkins.

Rubin, K. H. (2001). *The Play Observation Scale.* College Park: University of Maryland.

Rubin, K. H., Fein, G. G., & Vandenberg, B. (1983). Play. In E. M. Hetherington (Ed.) & P. H. Mussen (Series Ed.), *Handbook of child psychology: Vol. 4, Socialization, personality, and social development* (pp. 693–774). New York: Wiley.

Ruffino, A. G., Mistrett, S. G., Tomita, M., & Hajare, P. (2006). The Universal Design for Play Tool: Establishing validity & reliability. *Journal of Special Education Technology, 21*(4), 25–38.

Runco, M. A. (2007). *Creativity theories and themes: Research, development, and practice.* San Diego: Elsevier Academic Press.

Sakemiller, L. M ., & Nelson, D. L. (1998). Eliciting functional extension in prone through the use of a game. *American Journal of Occupational Therapy, 52*, 150–157.

Salonius-Pasternak, D., & Gelfond, H. (2005). The next level of research on electronic play: Potential benefits and contextual influences for children and adolescents. *Human Technology, 1*(1), 5–22.

Sandnabba, N. K., Santtila, P., Wannas, M., & Krook, K. (2003). Age and gender specific sexual behaviors in children. *Child Abuse & Neglect, 27*, 579–605.

Sandseter, E. B. (2007). *Risky play among four and five year-olds in preschool.* Vision into Practice CECDE International Conference. Retrieved February 15, 2007, from http://www.cecde.ie/english/conference_2007.php

Sapp, D. D. (1995). Creative problem-solving in art: A model for idea inception and image development. *Journal of Creative Behavior, 29*, 173–185.

Saracho, O. N. (1990). Preschool children's cognitive styles and their social orientations. *Perceptual and Motor Skills, 70* (3 Pt. 1), 915–921.

Saracho, O. N., & Spodek, B. (1998). Preschool children's cognitive play: A factor analysis. *International Journal of Early Childhood Education, 3*, 67–76.

Saunders, I., Sayer, M., & Goodale, A. (1999). The relationship between playfulness and coping in preschool children: A pilot study. *American Journal of Occupational Therapy, 53*, 221–226.

Scarlett, W. G., Naudeau, S., Salonius-Pasternak, D., & Ponte, I. (2005). *Children's play.* London: Sage.

Schaaf, R. C. (1990). Play behavior and occupational therapy. *American Journal of Occupational Therapy, 44*, 68–75.

Schaaf, R. C., Merrill, S. C., & Kinsella, N. (1987). Sensory integration and play behavior: A case study of the effectiveness of occupational therapy using sensory integrative techniques. *Occupational Therapy in Health Care, 4*(2), 61–75.

Schaaf, R. C., & Mulrooney, L.L. (1989). Occupational therapy in early intervention: A family-centered approach. *American Journal of Occupational Therapy, 43*, 745–754.

Schafer, G. E. (1994). Games of complexity: Reflections on play structure and play intervention. In J. Hellendoorn, R. van der Kooij, & B. Sutton-Smith (Eds.), *Play and intervention* (pp. 77–84). Albany: State University of New York Press.

Schell, B. (2003). Clinical reasoning: The basis of practice. In E. B. Crepeau, E. S. Cohn, & B. A. B Schell (Eds.), *Willard & Spackman's occupational therapy* (10th ed.). Philadelphia: Lippincott, Williams & Wilkins.

Schell, B. B, & Schell, J. W. (2008). *Clinical and professional reasoning in occupational therapy.* Philadelphia: Lippincott, Williams & Wilkins.

Schiller, F. (1875). *Essays, Aesthetical and Philosophical.* London: Bell and Sons.

Schlenz, K. C., Guthrie, M. R., & Dudgeon, B. (1995). Burnout in occupational therapists and physical therapists working in head injury rehabilitation. *American Journal of Occupational Therapy, 49*, 986–993.

Schoen, S., & Anderson, J. (1999). Neurodevelopmental treatment frame of reference. In P. Kramer & J. Hinojosa (Eds.), *Frames of reference for pediatric occupational therapy* (pp. 83–118). Philadelphia: Lippincott Williams & Wilkins.

Schor, E. L. (2003). Family pediatrics: Report of the task force on the family. *Pediatrics, 111,* 1541–71. Retrieved June 11, 2008 from http://pediatrics.aappublications.org/cgi/content/full/111/6/S1/1541

Schmid, T. (2004). Meanings of creativity within occupational therapy practice. *Australian Occupational Therapy Journal, 51*(2), 80–88.

Schneider, P., & Gearhart, M. (1988). The ecocultural niche of families with mentally retarded children: Evidence from mother-child interaction studies. *Journal of Applied Developmental Psychology, 9*, 85–106.

Schwartzberg, S. L. (1993). Therapeutic use of self. In H. L. Hopkins & H. D. Smith (Eds.), *Willard and Spackman's occupational therapy* (8th ed., pp. 269–274). Philadelphia: Lippincott.

Scott, D., & Willits, F. K. (1998) Adolescent and adult leisure patterns: A reassessment. *Journal of Leisure Research.* Retrieved July, 22, 2008, from http://findarticles.com/p/articles/mi_qa3702/is_199807/ai_n8784241

Servin, A., Bohlin, G., & Berlin, L. (1999). Sex differences in 1-, 3-, and 5-year-olds' toy-choice in a structured play-session. *Scandinavian Journal of Psychology, 40*, 43–48.

Shine, S., & Acosta, T. Y. (1999). The effect of the physical and social environment on parent-child interactions: A qualitative analysis of pretend play in a children's museum. In S. Reifel (Ed.), *Play & culture studies: Volume 2: Play contexts revisited* (pp. 123–139). Westport, CT: Ablex.

Sigafoos, J., Roberts-Pennell, D., & Graves, D. (1999). Longitudinal assessment of play and adaptive behavior in young children with developmental disabilities. *Research in Developmental Disabilities, 20*, 147–161.

Singer, D. G., & Singer, J. L. (1990). *The house of make believe: Children's play and the developing imagination.* Cambridge, MA: Harvard University Press.

Singer, D. G., & Singer, J. L. (2001). *Handbook of children and the media.* London: Sage.

Singer, D. G., & Singer, J. L. (2005). *Imagination and play in the electronic age.* Cambridge, MA: Harvard University Press.

Siviy, S. M. (1998). Neurobiological substrates of play behavior: Glimpses into the structure and function of mammalian playfulness. In M. Bekoff & J. A. Byers (Eds.), *Animal play: Evolutionary, comparative, and ecological perspectives* (pp. 221–242). New York: Cambridge University Press.

Skaines, N., Rodger, S., & Bundy, A. (2006). Playfulness in children with autistic disorder and their typically developing peers. *British Journal of Occupational Therapy, 69*, 505–512.

Skar, L. (2002). Disabled children's perceptions of technical aids, assistance and peers in play situations. *Scandinavian Journal of Caring Sciences, 16*(1), 27–33.

Skard, G., & Bundy, A. C. (2008). Test of playfulness. In L. D. Parham & L. S. Fazio (Eds.), *Play in occupational therapy for children* (2nd ed., pp. 71–93). St. Louis, MO: Mosby Elsevier.

Skellenger, A. C., & Hill, E. W. (1994). Effects of a shared teacher-child play intervention on the play skills of three young children who are blind. *Journal of Visual Impairment & Blindness, 88*, 433–445.

Skellenger, A. C., Rosenblum, L. P., & Jager, B. K. (1997). Behaviors of preschoolers with visual impairments in indoor play settings. *Journal of Visual Impairments and Blindness, 91*, 519–530.

Slade, A. (1987). A longitudinal study of maternal involvement and symbolic play during the toddler period. *Child Development, 58*, 367–375.

Smith, D. T. (2000). Parent-child interaction play assessment. In K. Gitlin-Weiner, A. Sandgrund, & C. Schafer (Eds.), *Play diagnosis and assessment* (2nd ed., pp. 340–370). New York: John Wiley & Sons.

Solomon, R., Necheles, J., Ferch, C., & Bruckman, D. (2007). Pilot study of a parent training program for young children with autism: The PLAY Project Home Consultation program. *Autism, 11*(3), 205–224. Retrieved from http://aut.sagepub.com/cgi/reprint/11/3/205

Sorce, J. F., & Emde, R. N. (1981). Mother's presence is not enough: Effect of emotional availability on infant exploration. *Developmental Psychology, 17*, 737–745.

Sparling, J. W., Walker, D. F., & Singdahlsen, J. (1984). Play techniques with neurologically impaired preschoolers. *American Journal of Occupational Therapy, 38*, 603–612.

Spencer, E. A. (1989). Toward a balance of work and play: Promotion of health and wellness. *Occupational Therapy in Health Care, 5*(4), 87–99.

Spencer, H. (1873). *The principles of psychology.* New York: D. Appleton and Co.

Spinka, M., Newberry, R. C., & Bekoff, M. (2001). Mammalian play: Training for the unexpected. *Quarterly Review of Biology, 76*, 141–168.

Spitzer, S. L. (1999). Dynamic systems theory: Relevance to the theory of sensory integration and the study of occupation. *AOTA Sensory Integration Special Interest Section Quarterly, 22*, 1–4.

Spitzer, S. L. (2003a). Using participant observation to study the meaning of occupations of young children with autism and other developmental disabilities. *American Journal of Occupational Therapy, 57*(1), 66–76.

Spitzer, S. L. (2003b). With and without words: Exploring occupation in relation to young children with autism. *Journal of Occupational Science, 10*(2), 67–79.

Spitzer, S. L. (2004). Common and uncommon daily activities in individuals with autism: Challenges and opportunities for supporting occupation. In H. Miller-Kuhaneck (Ed.), *Autism: A comprehensive occupational therapy approach* (2nd ed., pp. 83–106). Bethesda, MD: AOTA Press.

Spitzer, S. L. (2008). Play in children with autism: Structure and experience. In L. D. Parham & L. S. Fazio (Eds.), *Play in occupational therapy for children* (2nd ed., pp. 351–374). St. Louis, MO: Mosby Elsevier.

Spriegel, W. R., & Myers, C. E. (1953). *The writings of the Gilbreths.* Homewood, IL: Richard D. Irwin.

Staempfli, M. B. (2007). Adolescent playfulness, stress perception, coping and well being. *Journal of Leisure Research.* Retrieved July 20, 2008, from http://findarticles.com/p/articles/mi_qa3702/is_200707/ai_n21185992?tag=rel.res4

Stagnitti, K. (2007). *Child initiated pretend play assessment (ChIPPA)* [kit]. West Brunswick, Victoria, Australia: Co-ordinates Publications.

Stagnitti, K., & Unsworth, C. (2000). The importance of pretend play in child development: An occupational therapy perspective. *British Journal of Occupational Therapy, 63,* 121–127.

Stahmer, A. C. (1995). Teaching symbolic play skills to children with autism using pivotal response training. *Journal of Autism and Developmental Disorders, 25,* 123–141.

Steese, B. (2009). Pirates of the CariBOOTin': Following the map to shoe tying success. *ADVANCE for Occupational Therapy Practitioners, 25*(7), 29–30.

Stephenson, A. (2003). Physical risk-taking: Dangerous or endangered? *Early Years: An International Journal of Research and Development, 23,* 35–43.

Stern, D. N. (1974). Mother and infant at play: The dyadic interaction involving facial, vocal, and gaze behaviors. In M. Lewis & L. A. Rosenblum (Eds.), *The effect of the infant on its caregiver* (pp. 187–213). New York: John Wiley & Sons.

Sternberg, R. J. (2006). Stalking the elusive creativity quark: Toward a comprehensive theory of creativity. In P. Locher, C. Martindale, & L. Dorfman (Eds.), *New directions in aesthetics, creativity and the arts. Foundations and frontiers in aesthetics* (pp. 79–104). Amityville, NY: Baywood.

Stevenson, G. S. (1940). Mental hygiene of childhood. *Annals of the American Academy of Political and Social Science, 212,* 130–137.

Stout, J. (1988). Planning playgrounds for children with disabilities. *American Journal of Occupational Therapy, 42,* 653–657.

Strasburger, V. C. (2001). Children and TV advertising: Nowhere to run, nowhere to hide. *Journal of Developmental & Behavioral Pediatrics, 22,* 185.

Sturgess, J. (2003). A model describing play as a child-chosen activity—is this still valid in contemporary Australia? *Australian Occupational Therapy Journal, 50,* 104–108.

Suizzo, M., & Bornstein, M. H. (2006). French and European American child-mother play: Culture and gender considerations. *International Journal of Behavioral Development, 30,* 498–508.

Sutton-Smith, B. (1997). *The ambiguity of play.* Cambridge, MA: Harvard University Press.

Sutton-Smith, B., & Kelly-Byrne, D. (1984). The idealization of play. In P. K. Smith (Ed.), *Play in animals and humans* (pp. 305–321). Oxford, England: Basil Blackwell.

Takata, N. (1974). Play as a prescription. In M. Reilly (Ed.), *Play as exploratory learning* (pp. 209–246). Los Angeles: Sage.

Tanta, K. J., Deitz, J. C., White, O., & Billingsley, F. (2005). The effects of peer-play level on initiations and responses of preschool children with delayed play skills. *American Journal of Occupational Therapy, 59,* 437–445.

Taylor, F. W. (1904). Principles of scientific management. In H. F. Merrill (Ed.), *Classics in management* (pp. 82–116). New York: American Management Association.

Taylor, K., Menarchek-Fetkovich, M., & Day, C. (2000). The play history interview. In K. Gitlin-Weiner, A. Sandgrund, & C. Schafer (Eds.), *Play diagnosis and assessment* (2nd ed., pp 114–139). New York: John Wiley & Sons.

Taylor, R., & Peloquin, S. M. (2008, April). *Teaching the therapeutic use of self—the intentional relationship model.* Presentation at the annual conference of the American Occupational Therapy Association, Long Beach, CA.

Taylor, R. R. (2008). *The intentional relationship: Occupational therapy and use of self.* Philadelphia: F. A. Davis.

Taylor, R. R., Lee, S. W., Kielhofner, G., & Ketkar, M. (2009). Therapeutic use of self: A nationwide survey of practitioners' attitudes and experiences. *American Journal of Occupational Therapy, 63,* 198–207.

Terr, L. C., Deeney, J. M., Drell, M., Dodson, J. W., Gaensbauer, T. J., Massie, H., et al. (2007). Playful "moments" in psychotherapy (Clinical Perspectives). *Journal of the American Academy of Child and Adolescent Psychiatry, 45,* 604–614.

Thomas, N., & Smith, C. (2004). Developing play skills in children with autistic spectrum disorders. *Educational Psychology in Practice, 20,* 195–206.

Thompson, K. V. (1998). Self assessment in juvenile play. In M. Bekoff & J. A. Byers (Eds.), *Animal play: Evolutionary, comparative, and ecological perspectives* (pp. 183–204). New York: Cambridge University Press.

Thorne, B. (1993). *Gender play: Girls and boys in school.* New Brunswick, NJ: Rutgers University Press.

Thorp, D. M., Stahmer, A. C., & Schreibman, L. (1995). Effects of sociodramatic play training on children with autism. *Journal of Autism and Developmental Disorders, 25,* 265–282.

Tickle-Degnen, L. (2002). Client-centered practice, therapeutic relationship, and the use of research evidence. *American Journal of Occupational Therapy, 56,* 470–474.

Tietz, J., & Shine, S. (2001). The interaction of gender and play style in the development of gender segregation. In S. Reifel (Ed.), *Play & culture studies Volume 3: Theory in context and out* (pp. 131–146). Westport, CT: Ablex.

Toomey, M. (2003). Creativity: Access to the spirit through occupation. In M. A. McColl (Ed.), *Spirituality and occupational therapy* (pp. 181–192). Ottawa, Ontario, Canada: Canadian Association of Occupational Therapists.

Trevarthen, C. (1980). The foundations of intersubjectivity: Development of interpersonal and cooperative understanding in infants. In D. R. Olson (Ed.), *The social foundations of language and thought* (pp. 316–342). New York: W. W. Norton.

Trevlas, E., Grammatikopoulos, V., Tsigilis, N., & Zachopoulou, E. (2003). Evaluating playfulness: Construct validity of the children's playfulness scale. *Early Childhood Education Journal, 31,* 33–39.

United Nations. (1989). Convention on the rights of the child. Retrieved June 1, 2008 from http://www.unicef.org/crc

Universal Design for Play Project. (2005). *Universal design for play tool.* Retrieved July 8, 2008, from http://letsplay.buffalo.edu/UD/udp_tool.htm

van den Berg, C. L., Hol, T., Everts, H., Koolhaas, J. M., van Ree, J. M., & Spruijt, B. M. (1999). Play is indispensable for an adequate development of coping with social challenges in the rat. *Developmental Psychobiology, 34,* 129–138.

van Rheenen, D. (2001). Boys who play hopscotch: The historical divide of a gendered space. In S. Reifel (Ed.), *Play & culture studies Volume 3: Theory in context and out* (pp. 111–130). Westport, CT: Ablex.

van Tubbergen, M., Warschausky, S., Birnholz, J., & Baker, S. (2008). Choice beyond preference: Conceptualization and assessment of choice-making skills in children with significant impairments. *Rehabilitation Psychology, 53*(1), 93–100.

Vergeer, G., & MacRae, A. (1993). Therapeutic use of humor in occupational therapy. *American Journal of Occupational Therapy, 47,* 678–683.

Vismara, L. A., & Lyons, G. L. (2007). Using perseverative interests to elicit joint attention behaviors in young children with autism: Theoretical and clinical implications for understanding motivation. *Journal of Positive Behavior Interventions, 9,* 214–228.

Von Klitzing, K., Kelsay, K., Emde, R. N., Robinson, J., & Schmitz, S. (2000). Gender-specific characteristics of 5-year-olds' play narratives and associations with behavior ratings. *Journal of the American Academy of Child and Adolescent Psychiatry, 39,* 1017–1023.

Von Zuben, M., Crist, P., & Mayberry, W. (1991). A pilot study of differences in play behavior between children of low and middle socio-economic status. *American Journal of Occupational Therapy, 45,* 113–118.

Vygotsky, L. S. (1978). *Mind in society: The development of higher psychological processes.* Cambridge, MA: Harvard University Press.

Wall, S. M., Pickert, S. M., & Gibson, W. B. (1989). Fantasy play in 5- and 6-year-old children. *Journal of Psychology, 123,* 245–256.

Whaley, K. L., & Rubenstein, T. S. (1994). How toddlers "do" friendship: A descriptive analysis of naturally occurring friendships in a group child care setting. *Journal of Social and Personal Relationships, 11,* 383–400.

White, R. (1959). Motivation reconsidered: The concept of competence. *Psychological Review, 66,* 297–333.

Wikler, L., Wasow, M., & Hatfield, E. (1983). Seeking strengths in families of developmentally disabled children. *Social Work, 28,* 313–315.

Williams, D. (1992). *Nobody nowhere: The extraordinary autobiography of an autistic.* New York: Times Books.

Williams, S. E., & Matesi, D. V. (1988). Therapeutic intervention with an adapted toy. *American Journal of Occupational Therapy, 42,* 673–676.

Wiltz, N. W., & Fein, G. G. (2006). Play as children see it. In D. P. Fromberg & D. Bergen (Eds.), *Play from birth to twelve: Contexts, perspectives and meanings* (2nd ed., pp. 127–140). New York: Routledge.

Wing, L. (1995). Play is not the work of the child: Young children's perceptions of work and play. *Early Childhood Research Quarterly, 10,* 223–247.

Wittman, P., & Velde, B.P. (2002). Attaining cultural competence, critical thinking, and intellectual development: A challenge for occupational therapists. *American Journal of Occupational Therapy, 56,* 454–456.

Wolfberg, P. J., & Schuler, A. L. (1993). Integrated play groups: A model for promoting the social and cognitive dimensions of play in children with autism. *Journal of Autism and Developmental Disorders, 23,* 467–489.

Wright-St. Clair, V. (2001). Caring: The moral motivation for good occupational therapy practice. *Australian Occupational Therapy Journal, 48,* 187–199.

Yerxa, E. J. (1967). Authentic occupational therapy. The 1966 Eleanor Clark Slagle Lecture. *American Journal of Occupational Therapy, 21,* 1–9.

Zill, N., Winquist Nord, C., & Loomis, L. S. (1995). *Adolescent time use, risky behavior and outcomes: Executive summary.* Retrieved from http://aspe.hhs.gov/HSP/cyp/xstimuse.htm

Zuckerman, M. (1971). Dimensions of sensation seeking. *Journal of Consulting and Clinical Psychology, 36,* 45–52.

Photo Credits

Index